RELEASE YOUR INNER

WILD

The modern day women's guide to reconnecting with your
true Self; honouring your health, passion and power

DANA MAHON

◆ FriesenPress

Suite 300 - 990 Fort St
Victoria, BC, V8V 3K2
Canada

www.friesenpress.com

ISBN
978-1-5255-4997-7 (Hardcover)
978-1-5255-4998-4 (Paperback)
978-1-5255-4999-1 (eBook)

1. HEALTH & FITNESS, WOMEN'S HEALTH

Distributed to the trade by The Ingram Book Company

This book is dedicated to wild women everywhere,
and the ones who love them, but leave them wild.

INTRODUCTION

YOU, MY DEAR, ARE WONDERFULLY WILD

—

You are Human.
You are Divine.
You are Grace.

You are here to live your wild journey.
Create it. Work at it.

There is nothing you can't get through.
You are so strong.
You are so much more than you know.

Life is short. Life is hard. Life is a blessing. Life is an extraordinary experience.
And yes, life is messy. Enjoy and embrace the messy, imperfect, untidy you
in all your glory. Then get off your butt and get to work to create the life you
want and deserve, and *then* surrender and let it unfold.
Learn to become a witness.

Life is opportunity after opportunity after opportunity to grow, stretch,
emerge, learn, and become more of yourself than ever before.

Each opportunity can take you closer to your wild spirit. To your Inner Wild.

Every opportunity is here for the taking. Life is now.

From my deepest, most heartfelt place, I hope you enjoy this read, take something from it, and at the very least laugh a few times both at yourself and with me. Then I hope you make whatever shifts you need, in order to connect with and release your Inner Wild.

Om. Peace. Love.
With blessings and gratitude
Dana

RELEASE YOUR INNER WILD
BECOME YOUR WILDEST, STRONGEST,
BEST VERSION OF YOU

My wish for all people is this:

May you be healthy, happy, free, wild, alive, and well. May you be, seek, and discover as much love as you can stand—the kind that makes your heart explode with gratitude. May you fulfill your dreams and may you always remember that your precious, beautiful life is full of opportunity, to create the experiences you want, and to manifest your most heartfelt desires. May you always remember that this is *your* life, and the sooner you live your truth, the brighter you will shine and the brighter our world will become.

May you be open like a bud in the springtime. May you burn bright and hot like a wild fire. May you always know and remember your greatness.

And may you

release

your

Inner

Wild.

This content is not intended to be a substitute for professional medical advice, diagnosis, or treatment. It is for informational purposes only. Please always seek the advice of your physician or other qualified health provider with any questions you may have regarding a medical condition.

GETTING STARTED

Let's start at the beginning...

We all have a wild and an Inner Wild. In fact, we are born with them. They live in us. What is wild?

Wild—as it relates to a plant or animal—can be defined as: *living or growing in the natural environment; not domesticated or cultivated. A wild, free, natural state of existence.*

Wild—as it relates to people—can be defined as: *uncontrolled or unrestrained, especially in pursuit of pleasure.*

The latter, has in it the essence of being almost hedonistic or reckless, whereas when referring to animals or plants, Wild has the connotation of being free and effortless, raw and natural. Very interesting.

Wild—as it relates to human behaviour—can also be defined as: *passionately eager or enthusiastic.*

I love the distinction among these. You see, every one of us—yes, every single person on earth—has a natural instinct to be wild. It's in our blood. If you're not so sure about this, recall the last time you danced on the edge of your comfort zone, took a risk, or did something "risqué." Even if you were afraid, you likely experienced a feeling of liberation, excitement, and/or even exhilaration. If you're not the risk taking type and can't relate to that analogy, notice how you start to feel when you've been inside or have been sitting too long or are unable to move freely. How you likely feel the urge and even the need to move—this is your Wild. Humans need to be unrestricted on occasion; otherwise ... well, stuff can go sideways.

What if you were able to openly and fully celebrate your Wild without being fearful of it causing disruption, chaos, or disorder? Because let's face it, this is one of the reasons people contain or ignore their Wild, keeping it tucked away nice and safely.

Knowing that we can tune into our Wild without disorder ensuing, is key, because as you just read above, in nature there is order and there is balance. Nature is untamed, yes, but within that, there is order. Nature is Divinely designed. Plants are located within proximity of other plants for a reason. Animals know the rules of their environment and they honour them. Simply put, there is a sense of ease in the wild; it's a beautiful, non-overthinking, and natural way of being that flows. Humans have somehow managed to mess up that flow by taking something pure and habitual, adding in our egos, and causing a disturbance to something that is inherently and divinely perfect.

Before we can return to the flow, first we need to understand what it truly means to be Wild, because most of us really haven't a clue. Hear me out.

For the most part, we think wild means partying, indulging uncontrollably *in the pursuit of pleasure.* We associate it with heading to Vegas to drink our faces off, gamble, go to strip clubs, have promiscuous sex, and come home saying what happens there stays there. Guess what. That isn't Wild. That is escapism, distraction, and desperately seeking a release of the Inner

Wild. Yet there is a reason why it is perfectly socially acceptable for grown adults to engage in this behaviour and, even further, encourage and celebrate it as something to tout! This behaviour is quietly understood among those who go—and even those who don't, to a degree—because deep down we all know that it's human nature to want to bust out. It isn't necessarily respected, but there is this code among humans that somehow deems this behaviour tolerable, or at least not punishable. And yet somehow it is socially unacceptable to walk around barefoot or hug a tree. Things that actually represent the Wild. Again, very interesting.

After the adrenaline rush or temporary escape of Vegas wears off, the issues that were there before will still be there, and if we've behaved recklessly—or worse, harmed another—on top of the anticlimactic exhausted feelings, can also lie regret and depression, especially once "reality" sets in and we realize we're exactly where we've always been, only now we're quite possibly depleted physically, mentally, and financially. I'm using Vegas here as an example; not everyone does Vegas, I get it, but you get the point. Indulgence and hedonism are not what connect us to our Wild.

Another and perhaps more trendy example of being wild is spending thousands of dollars to travel far away from home and camp in the wilderness, where we run into the ocean naked under someone's guidance, light a fire, and dance wildly around it until dawn. Now this is in itself wild, there is no doubt. But make no mistake ... we don't need to spend money or go anywhere to find our Wild. The outdoors can assist ... sure, maybe. I found mine while sitting inside my cabin listening to the sound of my breath. Of course, you will find yours in your own way. I am just here reminding you that your Wild—well, she is with you, each and every breath that you take; she never leaves.

So it's no wonder we're a bit confused about how to honour and celebrate our Wild, because not only are we not taught how to nurture it, we're taught to conceal it or cover it up under the guise of partying or "letting go."

Once we understand that our Wild is deeply connected to our spirit and to the spirit of the Universe, we are in a much better position to honour it. Whoa—mind blowing, hey?

Wild is intuitive; it is not cerebral. It isn't something we overthink or decide to be because it's cool to be Wild. It is something we feel. It is a strength that we possess that we can turn to time and time again to lead the way. It is a part of us. It's the part that knows when we're ready to pounce, or retreat, or hide, or go-in for the kill, so to speak. Being Wild comes from a place of inner power and strength. It takes fearlessness, confidence, trust, and all-knowing. Wild is an inherent intelligence.

The Wild inside of us wants to play every now and then, be fed a piece of raw meat, and be given the freedom to take risks, within reason. It wants to be heard and acknowledged.

But in fairness, when do we learn that feeding our Wild is essential to our happiness and to our greatness? Oh, I know—when we're about to lose our crap, or worse, never, and that's a bit late, now, isn't it?

Some people lean into the notion of living instinctually, and some try to block it out. I use the word "try" because the truth is that we can't actually block out our Wild—not permanently anyway. We can only pretend to. Some people get so good at pretending that they actually live a life that bottles up this energy and it either erupts one day, or they never experience its full pleasure. Both are fairly unfortunate. Now, wherever you are on the spectrum of Wild awareness is perfect. You picked up this book for a reason, and I'm guessing it wasn't to learn how to tame your Wild. It was to reconnect with it—to embrace it and to release it out into the world!

MEETING YOUR INNER WILD

OK, so now that we've examined Wild a bit more closely, we will, within these pages, examine how you can acknowledge and honour both your Wild, and your Inner Wild—what they need in order to survive in a healthy, thriving environment, and then how you can consciously create that environment.

When we are connected to our Inner Wild, releasing it then becomes an act of service to ourselves to make space for new energy to come in, to release old or stagnant energy, and ultimately to heal.

Lots to think about, yes. But how much fun and how liberating!

I've tossed around a few things here. Wild and Inner Wild, both are entirely critical to you living your best life. So what *is* Inner Wild?

Your Inner Wild is your Wild with some added dimension. It is your Wild, yet even more subtle. Imagine digging down one more level. One more layer. Or perhaps several, to get to the seed, the innermost part of yourself. Your Inner Wild can be thought of as, or compared to, your untamed Spirit.

Your Inner Wild is who you are—when you are free, unencumbered, and unburdened. It is who you are when you are yourself, without pretending or masking. Your Inner Wild is your instinctively human Wild nature coupled with your own unique extraordinary essence, the most primal aspect of yourself. Your Inner Wild is who you were born to be.

I use both *Wild* and *Inner Wild* interchangeably on occasion depending on the context but you'll totally understand both references!

In order to discover, connect with, and release your Inner Wild, you first need to know who you are. Like really know. You need to be sure of who you are, unapologetically. Knowing yourself means not doubting who you are and certainly not seeking the permission of others in order to be the Divine creature that you were put on this earth to be. Over the course of your life, if you're doing "the inner work," the self-study, the personal development, the peeling back of the layers, the digging deep, you start to become crystal clear on who you are. You will see how with some practice and consistent high-vibe habits like moving your body, eating nourishing foods, participating in positive relationships, and removing toxins—both physical and otherwise—not only will you know yourself, you will know where to go next on your path, feeling centred, sure, grounded, confident, and excited to take the next step—whatever that is for you.

According to the ancient practice of yoga, we (humans) have what are called koshas—bodies, layers, or sheaths—and there are five. Picture those little Russian dolls for a moment, one inside another inside another. Starting at the gross layer, or sheath, is your physical body; moving inward to the breath or energetic body; inward again to the mental and emotional layer; next, the intellectual layer, where we exercise judgment, discernment, and intuition; and finally, to our innermost place, our bliss layer. It is here that I think of as my Inner Wild's home. Well, it floats, or dances, if you will, between the intellectual/intuitive layer and the bliss layer. Inner Wild is guided by intuition and also by Spirit.

In this book you will get to explore and travel along your path to discover where your Inner Wild lives. A more exciting, fulfilling journey to undertake I cannot even imagine. If you feel unclear about where your Inner Wild lives or what it needs, that's awesome. You will be clearer by the end of this book! Think of this time with me as an opportunity to meet yourself again in new ways.

A BIT ABOUT ME AND MY WILD

So thank you for noticing this book and, moreover, for noticing within yourself the desire for something, even if you're unsure of what that is. Thank you for recognizing your desire to connect more deeply with yourself, because, in fact, this is your life's work.

If you are like me, you know there is more to life than routine and mundaneness. You know you are meant for greatness, and you've decided it's time to uncover yours. Awesome.

As somewhat of a seeker, even in my early teenage years, I've picked up many books, read many inspirational quotes, explored non-traditional paths of healing, and adopted many practices, all with the intention of raising my vibe—in other words, building the capacity for a healthy, vibrant, confident woman to emerge; to realize my true purpose, and connect to Spirit or Source. There was such value in each and every one of these offerings, but I discovered over time that the one thing missing for me was the compilation of these amazing lessons.

In my brain and in my heart lie these lessons and discoveries, the things that inspired me and led me to my now. And while I would love to think I can recall and access them all, I must admit this likelihood is shaky at best. Some lessons really stuck, some I needed to re-read, and some I let drift. The reason I wrote this book was so that you can have access in one place and in an easy-to-read, portable compilation, all of the lessons I have learned both from experts and my personal life experiences. This way, when you need or want a refresher, you need not search through seven books—that is, if you can even remember what came from which one.

Here I share my most tried and true ways of cultivating personal wellness and spiritual evolution, self care, and, yes, reconnecting with my Inner Wild, in the hopes that even one of the ways will spark something in you to keep you moving forward on your path to wholeness and Wildness. Because let's face it, Wild sounds pretty fun, doesn't it?

Here's the cool thing: I offer a simultaneously soft and Wild approach to life. This is not a combo commonly explored, and it is one that truly nourishes the whole you.

You may be wondering, *Can I feel Wild and at ease at the same time?* Indeed you can. In fact, it is actually simple. For real. And it's all within your control.

Before we go further, you should know that I'm a real woman. I work. I do my own laundry (when I feel like it). I don't have a trainer or a chef. I don't have a housekeeper. I don't use fancy or expensive miracle products. I don't own a TV. I am not a millionaire, in case you're wondering, but I have yet to be in debt, and at any given time I always have the resources to pay my bills, play, go on vacations, and ensure I enjoy the life I have chosen to live. As I am writing this, I live in a small town on beautiful Vancouver Island in a 300-square foot suite above my yoga studio. Livin' the dream, as they say. I've had more, I've had less, but one thing I can say for sure is that at forty-five, I am healthier, happier, freer, and stronger in all the ways, bolder, glowy-er, more content, and more at peace and at ease than ever before.

I share this statement with the intention that you start to believe this is possible for you and then get out (or in there!) and make it happen.

You should also know that sharing my love for healthy, vibrant, Wild living is my greatest passion, and with passion sometimes comes fire, so please pardon and accept my fire. I offer it up humbly with the best of intentions. I pose certain questions and share specific examples to encourage everyone to get real. If we can't do that with and for ourselves while reading a book, then when can we? If you want to make changes, you need to acknowledge where you are, and at the end of the day, you're the only one you need to live with. Truly. So notice where you get triggered or reactive—I won't take it personally. It may mean there is something unresolved deep within you. It's all good. Get curious. It's called peeling back the onion. Besides, if I didn't provoke a wee little bit, this book would be boring AF.

I promise if you read the whole book, you'll find I certainly have opinions, but you'll also find I can be quite loving, passionate and compassionate, and am hell-bent on supporting you on your path to wellness and Wildness because the more people out there who are happy, healthy, Wild, and connected to Spirit, the better off the human race is. Agree?

TAPPING IN

So why did you pick up this book? My guess is that, like many people, you are seeking a solution. Perhaps you want to make a change. Perhaps you want to feel better. Perhaps you want to release your Inner Wild. I'm guessing that the word "Wild" was definitely a draw; otherwise, you may have skipped over it. Perhaps you are examining your life and wondering if you can feel more vibrant, powerful, resilient, and stronger—physically, mentally, and emotionally—and at the same time experience more ease, peace, and, yes, Wild freedom to be who you are, as you are; to be the real you, all of the time, not just on the weekend or when you're alone in your pjs pulling a full-scale Bridget Jones.

Within these pages you will find your solution, and not because it is a magic bullet. Quite the opposite. We'll examine ways in which to nourish and move your body that will create a sense of Wild intimacy with yourself (and I'm not referring to sex; I am referring to reconnecting with your temple, your skin, your senses, and remembering what it feels like to feel). We'll explore a more peaceful approach to life while practicing how to speak your truth and set boundaries, and how to enjoy the pleasures that over time you may have let fall away. I believe the practices in this book will reconnect you with what you already know deep within your Wildest Self, and then it is up to you to get to work. Yes, creating shifts in our lives requires effort, but I'm going out on a limb here and assuming that you're ready for it, because if you're reading this, you've been putting in effort somewhere, but it just isn't paying off how you'd liked or hoped, or perhaps it is misdirected effort (i.e. you feel like you're stuck or have reached a point where you're not sure where to go next). We've all been there.

Or hey, perhaps the cover simply caught your eye.

And now you're here. Exactly where you need to be.

And perhaps you need a reminder that you can do anything you want and you can have anything you desire. Consider this your reminder. I did it and so can you!

Through some invaluable lessons, I have learned how to be a better, kinder, more compassionate, grounded, and at the same time Wilder, freer, and stronger human. I have learned through some joyful as well as painful experiences how to reduce suffering and how to experience more ease, better health, and loads of abundance, both financially and energetically, as well as how to not only rediscover, but honour my Inner Wild. It was when I tapped into that Wild that I started living a life of freedom and contentment. And the freer I felt, the more I could nurture my Wild side. It became this beautiful cycle.

Contentment—let's take a moment to examine this word. It is often interpreted as a kind of uneventful satisfaction. Like, meh.

Wikipedia tells us that contentment is actually a "mental or emotional state of satisfaction that may be drawn from *being at ease* in one's situation, body, and mind." This, my friends, is what we as humans seek—satisfaction. Sometimes we seek happiness. Personally, I seek ease but not just any ol' ease. Ease in the body *and* mind. In my humble opinion, contentment is even "better" than happiness, since it feels more steady and less emotional. Emotions fluctuate. It is from a place of steadiness, contentment, and ease that life starts to feel really great. I am pleased to say that I experience this feeling of contentment every single day in some capacity regardless of life's ups and downs and despite stressors and unpredictable situations. The cool thing is that I wouldn't trade all the elation in the world for this feeling. Trust me when I say contentment is the goal most humans overlook.

I know you don't know me yet, but you *can* trust me. Ask anyone about my integrity. I teach yoga to kids. You can't be a fraud when you do that; those little buggers would see right through me.

You may not have been seeking contentment when you picked up this book, but it is something that will "just" happen over time if you pay attention and introduce some of these practices into your life. Some have been part of my life since my teens, and some are newly appointed practices that I really started to implement steadily in my late thirties and early forties. They are shockingly effective for cultivating feelings of peace, wellness and contentment. And yes, age is just a number. The reason I reference it is to reassure you that it doesn't matter how young or old you are in relation to creating the life you want. As the saying goes, it is never too early or too late to be whoever you want to be. People have said to me, "After you turn forty, everything starts to fall apart." To which I've replied, "Hell no. I am not participating in that program. Uh uh, no way, sista." Practical things like exercise and taking care of my body-temple will always be a priority, of course.

Add to that, speaking my truth, exercising boundaries, and taking care of #1, well there's no stopping me now. Fall apart? I think not.

What I'm getting at here is that it is our code of ethics, teaching people how we want to be treated, dumping self-limiting beliefs, and trusting the process of the Universe, that are powerful beyond measure when it comes to discovering our Inner Wild. Integrate these beliefs and I promise you will feel more connected to your Wild side than ever before.

Consider me your walking, living life experiment, who can prove beyond a shadow of a doubt that you can do and can have anything you choose. The suggestions and offerings I make are not complicated, and while they take some work, they are sooo rewarding. Some have instant pay-off and some take a bit more time, but the journey is delicious. As you reacquaint with your Inner Wild, your deepest place, and your true Self, life actually becomes more fun, more exciting, and at times unpredictable … and not in a scary, out-of-control way, but in a "Yeah, I created this" kinda way.

No matter where you are on your path, what age you are, whether you're an intro or extrovert, whether you identify as shy, bold, confident, insecure, or someone who feels anything but Wild and fun and free, you can reconnect with and release your Inner Wild, and in fact, you *must*. Connecting to that place deep within, discovering your Inner Wild, creating the life you want, doing things you love with passion and purpose – this is your responsibility. It is your job to do this work, because the world needs more of that energy. See, it is our responsibility while here on earth to raise the vibration of our planet. Let's stop wasting time trying to chase money, or working ourselves to death so that we can earn a pension cheque. I mean I get it, pensions are good too (smile) but think about this for a second, each of us has been gifted with this life. We don't just get to earn money, pay bills and die. There is work to be done. Spirit work. What is your gift? Are you using it? Are you sharing it? If so, amazing! If not, what can you do to start now, today? It doesn't have to mean quitting your job hoping money will just land in your lap. In fact it isn't about money at all. It is about finding something that makes you want to spring out of bed in the morning or stay up late because you are so motivated and driven to use your gifts, in service to others. Imagine if everyone created the opportunity to do what they love? Artists. Healers. Musicians. Teachers. Pilots. Tree Planters. Baristas. Car Mechanics. What if every person was doing exactly what they wanted to do and was amazing at it because they loved it? Because it was their gift. Imagine the frequency that would create?? So please, do your part, take a look at your gifts, tap into them and start sharing them, in ways big or small... and there are no small ways.

COMMITMENTS

—

Suggestions for Getting the Most Out of this Book

Let go of fear—it serves no purpose on this particular journey. You are safe.

Take what you need—leave what you don't.

Incorporate what you can now, plants seeds for later, review, re-water, reseed as needed. Last I checked, books don't go bad.

Give yourself space to read, process, digest, and apply these offerings.

Keep an open mind. Yes … open that puppy right up.

Believe that you can do anything you want. If you don't believe it yet, that's OK; refer to the point above.

Be gentle with yourself as you introduce these new concepts and practices. Refrain from judging or grading your integration, and then … notice when it's time to give yourself a butt-kick into action.

Find someone you can share this journey with—stay open to the possibility that this person may appear precisely when s/he is meant to. If you don't currently have a person you trust and with whom you want to share, it's all good. Besides, you can always share with me!

I share what has helped me over the last thirty-plus years to become my best, most amazing self, even when life was hard and I felt uninspired, defeated, exhausted, and at times even a bit hopeless. As humans I believe it is our duty to share with fellow humans what may, in fact, help them along their journeys. I am confident that the lessons I've learned and experiences I've had can help you, and who knows, perhaps even spare you some unnecessary pain and suffering. Wouldn't that be nice? And I sincerely hope you share back with me your experiences after reading this. I want to see you soar as you emerge into your Wildest, best self.

I wanted to share how I reconnected with my Inner Wild, and even more than that, how I started to release it out into the world. So. Much. Fun. P.S. When you release your Inner Wild, other people can't help but notice and they want in to the "club". What you do and how you do it makes a difference to the people around you.

I'll explain as we go.

Plus, you will save thousands, maybe even tens of thousands, of dollars that otherwise may have been spent on things that will never in the long run bring you lasting happiness or wellness. You can thank me later.

** So for the sentence you may have been waiting to read:

With some simple yet amazingly effective lifestyle and attitude adjustments,
you can have it all. True story! Freedom. Health. Peace. Sass.
Wellness. Ease. Wealth. Abundance. Confidence. Liberation.

HERE WE GO ...

Humans are animals. This we know. Over time we have evolved physically, technologically, and possibly mentally ... possibly. It is questionable, however, as to whether we have actually evolved emotionally, socially, or spiritually, or if we have become so disconnected from nature, our origins, and the wild, that we have in fact lost our way and even regressed. For as long as time has existed, humans have craved something about the wild—likely because it is where our roots lie and instinctively we know this and need this. In modern times it's like we want to be wild again but we've forgotten how. There is a deep yearning to let go, to be free and uncontained, and yet there is a fear of doing these very things. The further away we move from the wild, the more unfamiliar it becomes; the more unfamiliar, the more fearful...cycle. Get it?

The part of us that is highly intelligent beyond measure, sadly is the part we possibly, or even probably, ignore or neglect. It's OK, we all do it from time to time. Rest assured, though, that you *can* reconnect with your Inner Wild.

Some of the ways I offer are soft, some are more assertive, and some are likely to create discomfort. But guess what. That is where the most extraordinary things happen—outside of your comfort zone. You will discover how to give that Wild within you what it seeks, which is some attention, without causing a volcanic-like eruption to the rest of your life.

If there is one gem I wish for you to take from this book, it is that you don't need to go hogWILD in order to satisfy your Inner Wild. You don't need to become a different person either; hey, unless you want to. All you simply need to do is pay attention to when your Inner Wild is speaking to you, and then with your full attention, grace, and heart, listen.

Have you ever stopped and asked yourself what being Wild means to you? Grab a pen and paper. Perhaps you want to take notes or jot down your initial thoughts and feelings. You can revisit these questions at any time.

When was the last time you contemplated your Wild side?

What would "being Wild" feel like?

Would you rather be Wild or tame?

Have you ever taken a walk on the Wild side of life?

What was it like?

Wild and Free

Wet 'n Wild

Wild Child

Wild World

Born to be Wild

Walk on the Wild Side

Wild Thing

Into the Wild

Our Wildest Expectations

As we see above, there are countless expressions, song titles, movie names—each containing the word *Wild*. Wild has this sexy connotation that intrigues, attracts, and excites us; and then of course it scares us too. Sometimes we don't even know why we want to be Wild; we just know that we do, or at least we want to feel small bursts of it.

So let me ask: *What does your Wild need in order to survive in a healthy environment, and how can you consciously provide that?* This is the part where you pause again and write stuff down. While I can't answer every single thing for you I can certainly pose the questions. Of course throughout the book I share with you what has helped me create that healthy environment. Right now I am asking you.

This next question I can definitely answer.

How do we release our Inner Wild safely, especially if we've caged it for so long that it feels stuck or afraid to emerge, or on the other side of the spectrum ... what if it feels explosive?

Either way, the answer is the same. Slowly.

It starts with spending time with and getting to know the Inner Wild again and what it needs, getting quiet with it and meditating on it until you feel you've connected with it. It doesn't have to be a long, epic thing. I am not saying you need to sit for hours, weeks, months, and years to locate your Inner Wild. Over time, bit by bit, as you pay closer and closer attention, your Inner Wild will start to emerge, and you will greet it with an open mind and heart instead of trying to shove it back down to the depths of your soul. You will start to greet it like an old friend.

Meditating on your Inner Wild … this may sound contradictory. It's stabilizing and perhaps the opposite of Wild. I get it. But remember, there is order in the Wild. It is methodical. It makes sense.

When we are grounded, steady, and have our stuff at least somewhat together, we can choose our Wild—not in an overly planned way, but also not in an entirely random or reactive way. When we aren't grounded or steady, we become reckless, desperate, frustrated, and destructive. When we are deeply connected to our Wild, we can trust our intuition, inner intelligence, and instinct. Make sense?

We don't need to be all bull-in-a-china-shop about it. In fact, here's the coolest thing about knowing your Inner Wild—there is nothing sexier or more powerful than someone who knows who she is; who knows she can handle herself with grace, confidence, and a deep, profound connection to her Wild *and* doesn't need to prove it. Boom!

BADASS VERSUS SPIRITUAL BADASS

Notice how some people walk around calling themselves wild women, or badasses, or "someone who has a strong personality," and that these personas are often accompanied by aggression, anger, ego, and a "don't F with me" kind of attitude. I should mention here that I am no stranger to profanity. I have been dropping F-bombs for three-quarters of my life. But being a strong, wild woman isn't about being harsh, aggressive, or tough on the exterior.

The word "badass," for example, has made its way into our regular mainstream vocabulary in the last few years or so. Badass and Wild are often used together or in similar interchangeable contexts. It seems women more than anything want to be badasses; they want to be wild and free.

It seems there is a desire to a) strive toward this and b) think it is something that makes us better or cooler or stronger somehow.

I get it. I wanted that too!

Let's examine the word badass: Badass might be defined as a *tough, uncompromising, or intimidating person.*

I don't know about you, but this is not the vibration I wish to be or project. It feels somewhat stubborn and rigid. It butts up against the Yogic approach to life I have come to embrace, appreciate, practice, and teach.

I'd much rather be a *spiritual* badass, meaning, having an uncompromising approach regarding my values, sure, but knowing what I want and, rather than being intimidating, being welcoming. I choose to have a spiritual underlay to me that says, "If you come closer, not only will I not bite, I will feed your Wild." To me, being a spiritual badass says I possess such mad skills, intelligence, confidence, and capacity to speak truths, with respect, in ways that show independence, integrity, strength (toughness), and boundaries, that I don't need to tell everyone about it. I mean, sometimes I do (smile), but it is usually in the context of reminding people not to hide their own spiritual badass selves! But first, understanding that it is very much an internal practice.

To me, being a spiritual badass says I am committed to living my best life and I encourage you to do the same. I will even lift you up. What's cool about this is that there is no mistaking who you are, what's important to you, how you will be treated, and what you will allow into your energetic and physical space ... and at the same time you are a kind, compassionate, caring human. Living this way contributes to the Universal Sound; it inspires others to be their best, who then go inspire others to be the same. It's contagious; it's like the Tasmanian devil of goodness. If that isn't Wild, I don't know what is.

For the record, I don't need to be a badass at all. I simply need to know who I am, what I stand for, and how to create my own peace.

But good Lord, if you're restless and impatient and need to feel wild or badassy while you reconnect with your Inner Wild, then go get wild, old school! Go out into nature. Take your shoes and socks off. Get your feet dirty. Hell, get your body dirty. Jump in the cold river or ocean. Skinny dip. Feel the elements and the aliveness that is the wild. (do it for free!)

GETTING OUT OF YOUR OWN WAY
WORDS, INTENTION, & MINDSET

Here are some more questions for you:

What are some of your self-limiting beliefs? Write them down.

I can't achieve _____ because _____ …

I'll never get a promotion because _____ …

I will be single forever because _____ …

I can't lose weight or reach my fitness goals because _____ …

I'm destined to be broke because _____ …

Other _____ …

Whatever it is for you.

Now, how are your self-limiting beliefs and behaviours serving you? What are you getting out of being sick, tired, broke, unhappy, or single? How is your dis-ease serving you? Write it down.

Remember, these are beliefs, not truths. Recognize them as such and then choose new beliefs and actions accordingly. Write those down too.

Have you ever doubted your greatness? Have you ever let something stop you from taking that next step or following your heart? Have you ever stayed somewhere too long—a job, a relationship, a city—because you were afraid you'd fail if you left to do something bigger or better or different? Have you ever let the opinions of other people keep you small? Moreover, have you started to adopt that way of thinking and now find yourself actually believing it? Has someone's opinion of you become *your* opinion of you?

If you're human, then you probably answered yes to a few of these. I certainly have. But I was very careful not to dwell in this place.

I truly know in my heart, and believe with everything in me that I have the resources to make my life exactly what I want it to be. And so do you! You may not believe that in this moment, but it's true. You and I are no different in this way. Every single one of us can create our path exactly how we want. What is stopping you? If you say money or time, I call BS. We all have the same twenty-four hours in a day, and there is more than enough money circulating to support everyone's dreams.

So I ask you again: What is stopping you or slowing you down? Who is stopping you or slowing you down?

Fine, I'll give you the answer. You are actually the only one who can stop you, so yes, these were trick questions.

You are stopping you. Why?

Who do you want to attract? What are you attracting? Who and what are you *not* attracting because of your other choices and self-limiting beliefs?

How often do you get so wrapped up in your thoughts and emotions that you become them? Ever hear the expression, "What we think we become"? or "We become what we think about all day long"? We can become our thoughts if we repeat them enough times, because they start to become our story. So what we tell ourselves matters. What is your story?

What we say matters. How we say it matters. Why we say it matters. It all matters. Our cells understand the vibration of our thoughts, which often become words. I am not a scientist; remember that everything I am sharing is based on my personal experience.

Based on our personal experiences and history, we see and hear things through a very unique-to-us lens, and based on that lens, we respond. Somewhere in there is a message we tell ourselves about what all of our observances and experiences mean. We cannot always control the thoughts that enter our minds, although with practice we get better at this. But we can definitely control the thoughts that stay, the messages we give ourselves, and the meaning we attach to things.

Words matter; they carry energy. Whether we are focusing on "positive" or "negative" thoughts, we will attract that energy in kind.

When we start to replace negative self-talk with positive, and exchange self-limiting beliefs for self-affirming beliefs, amazing things to start to happen. It takes practice and consistency. It takes patience, especially if we are programmed to dwell in the negative or to habitually think about what's wrong versus what's awesome.

We need to genuinely believe that what or whom we want to attract is already available to us, and then we need to believe we deserve it and take action to make it happen. We are often so close to manifesting what we want, and then we go ahead and sabotage it. Like, WTF!? We give up before we've even tried or discovered if we can succeed, or we give up when we are sooo close to reaching our goal. Why? Because it is so much easier (so we think) to stay safe, small, and comfortable. But then we have to start all over again next time we're ready, so, really, this approach isn't easier at all.

Get out of your own way and watch what happens. Start walking around like the person who already has exactly what she wants. Try it. And then try it again. Try on the feeling of success, achievement, and strength; see how it fits. At first it may feel too tight or awkward; maybe it feels baggy and sloppy. You may be fidgeting or pulling. Over time as you adjust to the feeling, it will fit like a glove or a comfy flannel and leggings. Perfectly.

REAL-LIFE EXPERIENCE

In November 2017, I revisited one of my favourite practices that had been introduced to me the year prior—the Miracle Morning. Hal Elrod, a young fellow with an amazing story, wrote a book called *The Miracle Morning*. I will summarize it in a nutshell, although I still highly recommend the read. After several life-altering events, Hal found himself in a deep state of apathy and depression, in a financial mess, facing the end of his relationship, and in a health crisis. He began to study the habits of the most successful people in the world, and not just financially successful people; he was looking to get out of debt and back into the world a healthier, more resilient man. Hal discovered that there were six habits among the majority of successful people. What he hadn't yet come across was someone who did *all* six, all the time. So he tried them one morning, for one minute each, to start. Silence, Affirmation, Visualization, Exercise, Reading, and Scribing. Well, he didn't refer to them as these initially, but his wife helped him come up with a clever acronym: SAVERS. Needless to say, these daily rituals changed his life in immense ways.

If you want the full monty, get the book or watch a video, but the bottom line is this… when I decided to practice the MM (Miracle Morning) for thirty consecutive days, my life changed too. Fast and fiercely. Waking up early was key. Although it isn't one of the SAVERS per se, the idea was to practice all six rituals at an early hour, thirty to sixty minutes earlier than would be a typical wake-up time. In addition to the six SAVERS, waking up early, as he found, was also one of the practices of successful people. There is a unique silence early in the morning.

Now, no one is saying we need to wake up at five a.m. to have a rockin' life. At the end of the day, we need to find what works. This was Hal's recipe however, and so I followed. It had an amazing impact on my ability to advance in my business, motivate others, become a leader in new areas, and smash some goals straight out of the park. I wrote down and repeated out loud things like, *My new yoga studio is thriving so much that I need to add more classes to the schedule. I am attracting the most wonderful people and becoming the best at what I do. People's lives are changing, and I can hardly keep up with all of the new business! I never dreamed my businesses would grow this quickly!* I read this out loud every morning, loud and clear, with the feeling it was happening. I read it like I was on Broadway. I projected my voice. I held my head and lifted my chest. I believed it all!

My intention was that by the end of the thirty days, all of those things would be realities. Guess what. Yeah, yeah, I know you know. Of course all of those became realities! The power of words I believed in and trusted, and the belief in myself was everything.

A few years ago I read, and mad-loved, Jenn Sincero's book, *You Are a Badass*, (yes Badass) and her description of the word "faith" as, "belief in the not-yet-seen." Can I get an amen!? We need to believe in the not-yet-seen, like feel in our bones, in our hearts, in our cores that what we want we can have. We don't need to wait for anyone or anything. In fact, what we want is already out there, we simply need to attract it.

Not once during those thirty days of Miracle Mornings did I stop believing, stop reading, or stop shouting out what I wanted to have happen and what I knew I could achieve. On the days I felt like skipping the six a.m. wake, it wasn't because I didn't believe; I may have been feeling lazy, but then I thought, *Woman, you told a whole hell of a lot of people you were doing this and you have taken on the role of leader for this month. Get your ass up and walk your talk.* And so I did. And the magic continued to happen. I have incorporated this practice into my everyday life as a result of the shifts that took place when I explored it for the first time. Sometimes I am up at 6, sometimes 8, sometimes it is for thirty minutes sometimes it is for six, but each day I sit on that cushion, I get quiet, I visualize my dreams, I believe they are happening now, I read my affirmations out loud, and I write down my thoughts for that morning. Why would I dare mess with this formula? P.S. exercise can be as simple as one minute of jumping jacks or anything that wakes up your body.

RECAP

——

Words are energy and they matter. Pay close attention to how you use your words. Are you using them for good or for harm? Are you manifesting your dreams or further perpetuating a situation that doesn't serve you? When we use our thoughts and words to create momentum, action, and positivity, there are truly no limits to what we can attract and manifest.

Find a practice that serves and suits you, a daily (ideally morning) practice that nurtures your dreams and gives you even the slightest bit of dedicated time to choose your words for that day and to remind yourself of your greatness and that you can achieve whatever you desire. Believe in yourself and then start walking around like the boss that you are.

DAILY RITUALS

I am the first one to dislike too much routine, structure, and conformity. I see these as jails of sorts, so eventually I bust out. I do, however, love my rituals. Semantics perhaps, but with rituals I feel a sense of devotion. I enjoy the calmness they bring and the impact on my mental and physical well-being. I see them as liberating rather than restricting. They feed me. I see them as ways in which I evolve and raise my vibration, things I do for me in order to be my healthiest, most grounded self, not as something that keeps me small and rigid. No no.

I could argue that this is the most important and life-changing section of this book. Why? Because how we set up and close our day is ... well, it's everything really. Our lives are made up of days, made up of moments. Rituals, when set with intention and practiced with consistency, are powerful ways to creating the life you want.

When I first incorporated some of these, I never thought in a million years I'd still be practicing them ten years later, and I certainly never thought anyone would listen to me when I swore they were life changing. But they did (listen), and they are (life changing). If you don't believe me, ask my yoga students, and not just the ones who were *all Yogic* beforehand; ask the ones who had never stepped foot in a studio, were ashamed of their bodies, and were skeptical at best.

Start with one or two rituals and add more as time goes. Or jump in full tilt, your call! You da boss. Please note, the habits and rituals you are about to read don't have to take long nor do they require a big investment or extravagant tools.

Total time for all rituals combined: ten to fifteen minutes (excluding the SAVERS and the one which takes fifteen minutes or so—I recommend reserving that one for when you have time to enjoy it fully). You can spend as much or as little time on each of these as you wish. Pick the ones you want to start with; there is no right and no wrong. Some days you may have it in you for a longer meditation practice or a more in-depth gratitude practice. For me, it is about establishing consistent habits without overthinking or judging.

GRATITUDE PRACTICE: TOTAL TIME: APPROX ... ONE MINUTE

The first thing I do upon waking is place one hand on my heart and the other on my belly. I offer up gratitude. *Thank you, body, for waking me up yet one more time. Thank you, heart, for beating throughout the night. Thank you, breath, for feeding my body while I slept.*

How blessed am I to wake up each day as a healthy, vibrant, vital human being, with my limbs intact, not to mention my mind, and with the ability to go out there and create whatever I want.

I thank all the souls who bless my life, my protectors and angels and guides.

Waking up from a place of gratitude is a game changer right there. Waking up a cranky pants, moaning about the job you hate or the schedule you "have to" follow today is not living from gratitude. If you aren't feeling grateful, find something for which to be grateful ... health, family, home, breath, heat, water, job, whatever it is. Starting the day this way sets us up for an entirely different human experience.

This attitude—if you will, this mindset—of not only not taking things for granted but actually *feeling* thankful and blessed for all that we have and get to experience, is often overlooked, in my opinion, and certainly underrated. As the saying goes—if we look at what we don't have, we have nothing; if we look at what we have, we have everything.

I'm human, so on occasion upon waking I mess it all up, check my device for the time, and inadvertently start scrolling before practicing gratitude, and then I feel like a bit of a shmuck, but this is what I mean. These rituals aren't so rigid that if I forget one or don't do it, something bad happens. These aren't obsessive rituals. These are feel good, set-my-day-up-for-greatness rituals. I notice that the more I practice them daily, the more I notice when they aren't part of my daily experience, and the less awesome I feel. Awareness is such a gift. When I don't give thanks, it feels ... wrong somehow, and not from a judgment standpoint but from a feeling that something is missing. I don't feel as grounded, steady, or ready to start my day without practicing my rituals, so I'd much rather not miss them. This is a choice, not an obligation, and over time, one that I have truly come to enjoy.

INTENTION SETTING: TOTAL TIME: APPROX ...ONE MINUTE

Each morning we can choose to be easy, observe our emotions, and decide that whatever comes our way today is A-OK. Not because everything that comes our way is A-OK, but because we choose to respond that way. This does not mean suppressing our feelings or allowing in abusive, invasive, or negative experiences without correcting or addressing them. Rather, it is about not letting those things or experiences determine how we will feel, and not allowing them to steal our peace. At least not long-term. We have moments where we get wrapped up, yes. Again, I am talking about not dwelling in those places.

When we wake up we can choose how we want to feel, and we can choose our intention for the day. This way, if the day starts going "off-course," we can bring our awareness back to this conscious choice we've made. When we choose how to start our day and what we want to bring into it, we can go out and create those things, but first we have to choose. If we don't … well then, we don't, and instead we're at the mercy of how someone else decided his or her day will go and what they need from us to make that happen. In other words, we get derailed and drawn away from our purpose and into someone else's.

If we don't choose our priorities and our action plan for the day, we end up involved in other plans that are not designed to get us closer to our goals. So we are either a) "simply" not getting our shit done and/or b) helping someone else get theirs done. We need to have goals so that we can create the life we want. If we don't, we are just zombies running around meeting other people's needs. Take charge of your day and ultimately your life with a morning routine to set intention, and then set your evening or nighttime intention to cultivate feelings of gratitude, well-being, and ease before you go to sleep and do it all over again in the morning.

SELF-CARE RITUALS

There is great power in incorporating daily practices of self-care, using the power of our own body and breath and nature's medicines to take care of all of our bodily systems.

Some people turn to shamans, a medicine man, or someone they trust deeply to bring healing and wellness into their lives. The reason is because those healers are deeply connected with nature and the wild. They are both intuitive and experienced, and they have a connection with the wild that many can't comprehend. The ancient rituals of Indigenous peoples are what preserve cultures and keep traditional practices alive. More and more people are turning to these wise healers because what people are seeking cannot be found in the modern world.

The connection between our physical and emotional health is undeniable, of course. What I love so much about the body is its power to heal itself when we provide the conditions for it. This means consistently supporting all of our systems in a variety of ways to maximize their efficiency, and not expecting each one to perform miracles under duress or stress. Day-to-day support of our bodies and minds, i.e. treating them how they deserve to be treated, like the homes that they are, not only feels good but sets us up for lasting health and vitality. If we aren't taking care, then what's the point really?

One of the most nourishing and ritualistic practices of self-care is known as Ayurveda, or the Knowledge of Life. Ayurveda, Yoga's sister science has also been referred to as the Science of Longevity. It is a lifestyle, a way of living in accordance with nature and the seasons and our own unique constitution, to bring the body and mind into a state of homeostasis, or balance. Using a comprehensive approach especially by emphasizing diet, herbal remedies, exercise, meditation, breathing, and physical therapy, Ayurveda is as beautiful as it is ancient and holistic. Here is a list of some of my most beloved Ayurvedic, and other daily rituals, which in yoga are called dinacharya.

MORNING

1. **Tongue Scraping. Yes, you read correctly. Total time: twenty to thirty seconds.**
   I can safely say that for the last ten years I have probably not missed more than five days of scraping my tongue. Once you introduce this practice there's no going back. Ask any of my yoga students who are now avid tongue scrapers.

   What is it and why do we do it?

   See, during the night the body produces bacteria, dead cells, fungi, and debris … sounds delish, yeah. These form at the back of the throat and then coat the tongue in the body's attempt to expel them. How brilliant. Now think about waking up and either guzzling a big glass of water or, worse, coffee, tea, or consuming food *before* helping the body complete the natural process it has already started. Tongue scraping, more effective and comfortable than brushing the tongue (gag), completes this process by removing what has built up, eliminating it from the body. Side note, gagging causes the eyes to water and actually helps to cleanse the eye balls so isn't necessarily a bad thing! Tongue scraping also activates our digestive system preparing our bodies for water and food.

Here are the five easy steps:

- Get yourself a scraper made from tin, copper, silver or brass. I confess mine is plastic and I have been using the same one since Yoga training in 2009. Don't judge me (smile). Scrapers are most often available at health food stores.
- In the morning upon waking, walk your ass to the bathroom.
- Scrapers have a little v-tip or a slightly more jagged ridge on one side of the U-shaped tool. Place the tongue scraper toward the back of the throat, with this side pointing down. If you have a strong gag reflex, feel free to start midway until you get used to it. The farther back you get eventually, the better, because the gunk starts back there, but there's no need to choke yourself or be aggressive. Remember, this is a self-care practice.
- Gently pull the scraper forward. I like to do ten or fifteen pulls, but in the beginning it may be less, and there is no real right or wrong or exact. You will see a whitish or yellowish film come off, depending on what you ate the day before, or more specifically closer to bed time.
- Rinse and clean the scraper. I run mine under hot water and place it back in a cup facing up. You may want to soak it in hot water with an essential oil such as lime or lemon for cleansing. Boom. Done. Almost coffee time.

2. **Morning Water. Total time: less than one minute or however long it takes you to drink a glass of room-temperature water.**

After my tongue is clean, I hydrate my body and cells with water. I often add a drop of a cleansing essential oil specifically formulated to aid in flushing my kidneys and liver and to support my system in preparing for the day; that or I squeeze in some fresh lemon juice. Side note: lemon, while acidic in taste, has an alkalizing effect when it enters the body. The only thing I like to mention is that while drinking it first thing is great, sipping on it all day can be hard on the enamel.

Because dis-ease flourishes in an acidic environment, it is important to alkalize the body, and morning is the perfect time to do this. We can alkalize water by adding ginger, lemon, mint, and cucumber. Adding these to a pitcher and letting the water soak up these nutrients alkalizes the water. If you live in a place where the water isn't the best, you may opt to boil, aerate and let it cool before drinking it.

I don't feel right about enjoying my coffee until I have watered (fed) my organs and set them up for success in all of the ways that they will need in order to perform optimally. I feel the water moving into my body to all of the spaces that need it. I imagine a river running through all sorts of rocks and crevices, touching, hydrating, and nourishing all of the places along the way.

Almost coffee time. Now is where I might add in my SAVERS but the order is up to you!

3. **Oil Pulling. Total time: two to five minutes to start.**
    An ancient Ayurvedic practice, oil pulling is said to support oral health, strengthen gums, remove bacteria from the mouth and gums, and even whiten teeth! Practiced with coconut or other oils like sesame or avocado, oil pulling involves swishing a teaspoon or tablespoon of oil for anywhere from two to twenty minutes. Working your way up may take time, and once you get the groove time flies. I prefer coconut as it has a natural foaming quality and swishes so nicely, as well as brightens my teeth. Add a drop of peppermint, clove, frankincense, tea tree, or any other pure, food-grade essential oil that you are drawn to, and swish while you boil water for tea or coffee, or as you tidy up the bathroom, sit in the sun, sit in meditation and focus on the act of swishing, write your to-do list for the day, make the kids' lunches … you get the drift. Do whatever you might otherwise do in the morning, and then, spit, ideally into a garbage versus a sink to prevent clogging. Be careful not to swallow the gunk you've just removed from your mouth. Spit. Rinse. Spit. Rinse. Then brush as normal. This will leave your mouth feeling squeaky clean, vibrant, and healthy.
    (You may also switch up the order of #2 and #3).

4. **COFFEE TIME! (Well, at least at this point it is for me.) Total time: However long you want!**
    In my home this is a ritual unto itself. In February of 2017, I went from being a tea-drinking, coffee-loathing human to a pretty-much-obsessed tea-drinker-turned-barista annoyingly-in-love-with-coffee-documentary-watching-social-media-posting-coffee maniac/lover. Yeah, it was weird. Why am I mentioning this? Because it has become a daily experience that I look forward to. After I've given thanks for waking yet another day, planted my feet on the ground, scraped my tongue, swished oil in my mouth, and then enjoyed some life-giving water, (sounds like a lot, but as you can see it can be like five minutes tops), I proceed to enjoy the art of making my espresso. Whatever your morning "elixir" is (mine is juice a few times a week but always a coffee with frothed cream!), the invitation here is to make a ceremony out of it. Even if it is a twenty second ceremony where you close

your eyes and inhale the aroma. Enjoying your pleasures is critical to ensuring that your mental and spiritual fires are stoked.

5. **Dry Skin Brushing. Total time: one to two minutes.**

Brushing the skin in a particular pattern with a dry brush, usually before showering, helps wake up the lymphatic and circulatory systems. The skin is typically brushed toward the centre of the body, starting with the bottoms of the feet working up the legs and brushing each section of the body ten times using gentle upward, long, smooth strokes. Repeat the same process with the arms, starting with the backs of the hands and brushing upward toward the armpits and heart. On the stomach, back and face, should you choose, use a circular, gentle, clockwise motion. Your skin will be exfoliated, and this simple act of dry brushing will leave you feeling energized and invigorated.

6. **Contrast Showers. Total time: one to two minutes during the last moments of your shower.**

At the end of your presumably warm or hot shower, alternate between cold and warm water. Go as cold as you can handle, alternating with the hot cycle running three times as long as the cold, and then switch back and forth a few times, finishing with cold. Not only does it wake you up, yikes, it increases circulation and blood flow, increases energy, keeps the skin and hair healthy, and is a fantastic and energizing way to start the day. I typically do this during my morning versus evening showers.

7. **Aromatherapy. All the time and everywhere.**

I could probably write an entire book just on the benefits of aromatherapy alone. Hmmm, not a bad idea. Ok, but for now I will say this—for more than 20 years, pure, potent and powerful essential oils have been my go-to remedy for pretty much everything from a cut or wound to menstrual cramps to a sore throat to managing anxiety to insomnia and literally anything in between. I refer to them in more detail later on where I talk about weekly rituals, but needless to say I literally can't imagine having the level of peace, health, stability, comfort and wellness without these gifts of Mother Earth. I never start or end my day without them, whether in my diffuser, on my wrists or back of the neck, in my diffuser necklace that I never take off, in my bag (I always carry a minimum of five roller bottles), in my bath or shower, in my shampoo, in my car in a spritz bottle, or just a few drops run through my hair. I feel blessed beyond measure to have access to these miracles that nature provides for us and I know on my deepest level that they are the reason I feel so darn good every day.

8. **Journaling. Total time: one to infinite minutes.**

The act of writing has been and continues to be a gift that is hard to explain until one experiences its benefits. I started my first journal when I was in my teens. It isn't something I can say I do with a hundred percent consistency or diligence. We are not perfect beings. I started journaling as a way to simply dump my thoughts. I have several on the go, and what I love about this act is that nothing is ever wrong. It is an extraordinary way to make space in the mind, to take a good close look at your roadblocks, to see what may be causing you to feel stuck, and also to see, in fact, how far you've come and to celebrate that progress. I quite enjoy reading past entries, either from way back or even a day prior. It is often humorous, at times upsetting, and mostly surprising how "in it" we can be at any given moment and yet in many cases how swiftly that intensity can pass. What a wonderful way to witness the impermanence of emotions. It gives us faith to believe that we will be and in fact always are OK. Sometimes I journal for one minute and sometimes my hand keeps going and it's ten or twenty minutes. There is no formula. When the mind is done, the hand stops. It's simple, really.

9. **Connect to Spirit. Total time: two minutes.**

On occasion I pull from my goddess oracle deck. I reconnect with that which is sacred—my divine feminine. I find her, I feel her, I thank her, I pray to her, I honour her. Truth? We are never not connected to Spirit; we simply need to remember this, and so this short ceremonial act helps me. Every woman needs a goddess deck whether she knows it yet or not.

10. **Deciding to Be a Good Human. Total time: five seconds.**

Yes, this is a ritual, consciously choosing to do good. Each day we can wake up with the intention to be good people and to reach some goals, or, at the very least not be shitty people. Deciding to be a good person feels good.

11. **Meditation. Total time: one minute-plus.**

As I talked about in the section earlier on mindset, one of the most powerful things you can do for yourself is learn how to manage your mind so that it doesn't manage you. One of the most effective ways to do that is through meditation. We have the ability to train our minds, yet how amazing is it that so many of us don't practice it. It seems daunting and pointless because the mind jumps around, I get it. But what I teach the kids is that the reason we spend time cultivating a calm mind and awareness of our breath is so that we can recognize when we aren't calm or aware, and then we can bring ourselves back to that peaceful state more and more often.

Meditation is a practice involving a single-pointed focus on something like an image, thought, phrase, syllable, word, or sound (mantra), which takes us out of our heads, bringing about feelings of calm and mental clarity. The studies around meditation are endless and all point back to the same conclusion. Meditation changes the brain. When we meditate, we are able to change the way our mind perceives emotions. When we meditate, we are able to manage the part of our brain responsible for fear, anxiety, and stress—the emotions and responses that plague millions of people every moment of every day because so many of us are not aware that we can actually turn that shit around, simply by noticing and then making the conscious choice to shift it. Through intention setting and meditation, even a few moments practiced consistently each day, we have the ability to change our daily experiences. Amazing.

It is important to be quiet and feel what we feel. It is here in the quiet that we can watch things settle. Often we want to escape and purge our thoughts or anxieties before we have even sat with them long enough to understand them. They are there to teach us something and they will keep arising until we learn from them. When we sit with our stuff first and let it defuse, even just a bit, in a matter of minutes the intensity of emotion often changes. It is really only in the quiet moments that we get the opportunity to witness and experience that. It helps us understand and truly believe that we have the power to manage how we feel; we just need to be willing to sit with stuff first. Here we notice physiologically, mentally, and emotionally the intensity of our thoughts and emotions. It is also here where we witness the intensity drop. It is a liberating experience and it teaches us how to manage the mind before it manages us. Once we do it a few times it is less frightening to sit with our thoughts and emotions, and this is what builds our capacity. Please please please before reaching for a distraction, try it. It is so empowering to come out on the other side of fear, stronger and bolder.

NIGHT

Night-time rituals are like the bookends on a blessed day. Even on the days that don't feel so blessed, there is always opportunity for, yes, gratitude, and also for some feel-good stuff, whatever you need to do to conclude the day and create some positivity before drifting off to slumber.

For me, night rituals are brushing and flossing the ol' teeth, washing my face (actually using a facecloth with warm water) to remove any dust or pollutants, putting on my favourite face oil, diffusing a beautiful and restful essential oil blend, and whatever else may be fitting for that day. An evening bath is a lovely way to unwind, or enjoying some herbal tea with turmeric and black pepper can support the immune system while at the same time preparing the body for rest. There are so many beautiful ways to honour the end of a day.

Sometimes I will apply oils to my feet and then put on cozy socks, especially if I need extra grounding that day. I find reading or thinking about something positive as my last cerebral effort is always nice. Sometimes it's listening to a mantra or a recording designed to support me in manifesting my dreams, like Yoga Nidra; a systematic full body and mind technique that relaxes the body, relieves stress and clears the mind. I am not here to direct your rituals but rather share how much of a difference they can make on your wellness journey should you wish to adopt them. I would love to hear what you come up with. Whatever it is, creating a nighttime ritual rooted in wellness, self-care, and love goes a long, long way.

WEEKLY

Weekly Self Massage: And yes, this is a bit of a longer practice. Total time: fifteen to twenty minutes if you have it, which is why it isn't necessarily a daily practice, but if you have the time I dare you not to get hooked.

In the Ayurvedic practice, there is a massage technique that can be self-administered or performed by a practitioner, called abyhangha, meaning massaging the body's limbs or "glowing body." It is performed by first finding an oil that works best for your constitution, and if you don't know what the heck I'm talking about, just pick one you like. If you tend to be fiery or if it's summertime, coconut oil is nice and cooling. If you tend to feel cool or if it's winter, almond or sesame is nice. Apricot oil is also lovely. If you need or prefer something a bit heavier, jojoba (pronounced huh-ho-bah) oil is a nice choice as well. Firstly, the oil is gently warmed. I like to place my bottle inside a glass jar or stainless pot containing hot water and let it sit for several minutes until it is warmed through. To this oil I add essential oils.

There is nothing more wild than tapping into nature and accessing the plant essences that have been used for thousands of years in order to promote wellness, reduce dis-ease, and to ground ourselves.

Essential oils have been around since there were plants to grow and harvest and use. When we get in touch with our bodies, we tend to gravitate to the medicines that the body needs, because the body is so highly intelligent, it knows. Every second, millions of cells die and are replaced. So we are literally constantly changing—of course, we need to pay attention and support ourselves as the body changes and moves through different stages: cedarwood, bergamot, lavender, frankincense for calming; peppermint, rosemary, lemon for energizing; wild orange, lime for uplifting; cardamom, eucalyptus, black pepper for respiratory support. And on it goes.

The time of year and what I am experiencing emotionally and physically helps me determine whether I am in need of something invigorating, calming, soothing, earthy, grounding, or uplifting. Next: I get naked and I start applying. Top to bottom without missing a spot. I apply the warm oil gently in a circular motion—to my scalp, my entire face, behind my ears, front and back of my neck, shoulders, underarms, chest, arms, breasts, over my heart, torso, front and back, hips, butt, and I work my way down to the soles of my feet and then in between the toes! This is an external application only, so I am mindful not to apply internally or into orifices. The heat from the warm oil and my hands increases circulation and blood flow, helping to activate the lymphatic system. The oils, of course, enter the body through the skin, as well as infuse the tissues, hydrating and nourishing them deeply. It is a brilliant way to practice self-care, to examine and inspect the body, and to get in touch with ourselves through the senses of touch and smell. It is an opportunity to be intimate with yourself. Where does your body feel free and easy, where does it feel tight and restricted, perhaps even guarded? The art of this massage is in the time and intention. It doesn't have to take your whole morning, but whatever time you do set aside, be present. Leave your phone in another room and connect with yourself. Maybe this is something you do once a week or once a month, but whatever it is, let it be your time. If it's going to be rushed, perhaps a different time would be more ideal.

I let the essential oils and whichever body oil I choose, soak in for as long as I can (fifteen to twenty minutes where possible). I'll read something inspiring, fold my laundry, write in my journal, or do whatever, and then I shower in warm water. I use soap in the shower for my lady bits, but I don't soap off the luxurious oils I've just applied. I let them continue to do their work all day. What an experience it is. After the shower I pat my skin dry. The only thing I apply afterward is some of my favourite nourishing natural body butter. I don't really need it to hydrate my skin on these self-massage days, but I love the aroma and what it does for my soul. My skin loves it too. I use a simple but gorgeous face cream that leaves my skin looking youthful, glowing, and radiant. This is my "beauty" routine. You can decide for yourself if it's something worth following. Simple and so enjoyable. You will feel like you've just left the spa and truly taken care of yourself. And you have. By the way, if you decide to get practical during this process you don't need shaving cream if you're a shaver, because the oil takes care of that.

I have been a natural girl since I was teenager and worked my first "real" job at a natural body-care store where I learned about the rarity of rose oil, and how peppermint, when applied to my temples or back of the neck could reduce or eliminate a headache. Now I know the power of aromatics and how for example lavender sniffed straight out of the empty bottle in my shower when I feel tense or anxious, or lime when I feel grumpy, are actually ways to invite in wellness and ease.

I am grateful for so many of the rituals that were introduced to me by way of Yoga and Ayurveda. Each one has impacted my life in a powerful and extraordinary way.

RECAP

—

Enjoying morning and evening rituals are a powerful way to take care of ourselves. Rituals allow us the time to check in, connect with our mental and emotional state, and prioritize our well-being, even if just for a few moments. Rituals bring with them a sense of comfort, stability, and grounding. Even the seemingly most minor ritual when practiced regularly can cultivate deep, meaningful, and long-lasting effects. Supporting our systems in all the ways is essential (no pun intended) to our overall well-being. It is only through consistent practice and healthy habits that we create a healthy vessel. Inside and out. Plant essences can be used to support our mental, emotional, physical, and spiritual bodies. It is an extraordinarily delicious way to practice self-care and develop a natural lifestyle that will bring you infinite pleasure and enjoyment. And it's super fun to be your own alchemist!

MOVE YOUR WILD BODY

(Spoken by a yoga teacher, so pardon my mini yoga training and most passionate, in-depth description and invitation for how to practice. I cannot help myself!)

We all know that our bodies are designed to move, not sit, at least not for extended periods. Whatever way you choose to move is perfect. As long as you enjoy it, you are benefiting. Some resistance training is great for building or maintaining lean muscle, which nicely keeps our muscular body in place, upright, and strong. Lean muscle keeps our internal furnace (metabolism) stoked and keeps the fat burning at a nice, even pace. Nothing crazy required, just something that creates resistance.

I prefer exercise that uses my body weight, like squats, lunges, push-ups ... things that use resistance but that don't require a gym or anything fancy shmancy. Whatever is sustainable is going to be the winner. I also like spurts, like fifteen-minute rounds. No big commitments. Gypsy souls don't like to be tied down (wink).

OK, so that is my obligatory "exercise for fifteen minutes a day" spiel, because tried and true it is good for our bodies and amazing for our mental and emotional health.

Here's the other deal.

When we move the body consistently over time, amazing things start to happen. Through movement and intentional breath (yoga, for example), we bring energy and vitality to parts of ourselves that may have otherwise been dormant or less vital. We open up our energy centres, or chakras, and if you don't believe they are real (wink) you can look at a Western/Eastern science diagram and see that the third eye relates to the pituitary and pineal glands, the heart chakra is the space where the heart lies, the throat chakra is found where the thyroid gland lies, etc...

During a yoga practice, "stale" energy moves, which is why it isn't uncommon for people to be moved to tears during or following a class. This is how we release the Inner Wild—by giving it space to emerge.

In my thirties I began my exploration of yoga. And yes, I know, why is it that when we talk about exercise in general, we say, "I started running," or "I took up kick boxing," but when we talk about yoga it is an "exploration"? Well, it just is. It is soooo much more than a form of exercise—in fact, the movement piece is only one-eighth of yoga. I included it in this section however because it is a brilliant way to move the body, and that's what I'm talking about here.

Yoga gets our circulation flowing, challenges our balance, strength, and flexibility and with practice becomes meditative and fluid. It can be practiced in classes, obviously, and also solo for free, and it is a wonderful way to get curious about your body. Yoga invites us to feel the inner workings of our bodies, and through gentle adjustments, we feel sensations in the most interesting of ways. Tendons, ligaments, and muscles that don't typically get used suddenly speak to us, and then we use our breath to stay in the experience without reacting. The most subtle movements can change an entire experience in the body. All we need to do is pay attention and notice. Over time, our bodies and minds open, expand, and become more supple. We become less prone to injury … of course, when practicing mindfully and within one's capacity.

LITTLE STORY

If you're wondering, yoga and I did not have a love-at-first-flow experience. Not even close. I went to my first class when I was about twenty-something, having no clue or expectation of what it would be like. I was shocked and frankly quite upset to learn that the sun salutation had no end. It literally went on forever. Actually. I had no guidance and certainly no one teaching me that yoga was controlling the thought waves of the mind. Had I known that, perhaps I wouldn't have been so obsessed with hurting the teacher. That was my last class for about five years. I stuck to teaching aquafit to the seniors in the warm pool at that same community centre. For whatever reason, years later I decided to attend a yoga class one day while figuring out what to do with my sorry, unemployed ass. After calling off my wedding, I moved back to Vancouver (2002-ish) with a hockey bag of my possessions in tow, along with a leap of faith, a hope, and a prayer. Well, something like that. I get into this story a bit further on in the book. Anyway, I had time on my hands, a very busy mind, and no money to burn. I lived down the street from a super-cool yoga studio on Commercial Drive, so even when you're unemployed with no plans, $15 for a class is somehow doable.

What a vastly different experience this class was from the never-ending sun salutation/ evil-thoughts-about-the-teacher, prior experience. This one was about quieting my mind, and someone actually explained this. The space felt nurturing and healthy. There I was, in my yoga pants with my positive attitude, wanting to learn everything I could, knowing in those moments that I had lifetimes of learning to get it "right," but I was hell-bent on travelling the path. I knew right then and there that yoga would be a life-changer and a significant part of my life. I moved six times in fifteen years with my then-partner, and each time I found a nearby studio and continued my practice. I took my mat on vacations to Mexico and Hawaii, and it was then that I knew in my deepest place that yoga would forever be a part of me. A couple of years later I purchased a little book called *1001 Pearls of Yogic Wisdom*. It was a little pocket book and basically a mini yoga teacher-training (YTT). I read it over and over. I took it on my summer boating vacations. I immersed myself. I learned the Sanskrit words for postures. I studied the philosophy that made so much sense. Now this was a practice I could get behind. Mentally, I felt relaxed; physically, I felt strong; emotionally and spiritually, I felt connected for the first time in a long time.

I finally made the choice to enroll in a six-month YTT program, through a community college. Teachers were independent and each had an extensive history and background in practicing and teaching yoga. The program was every other weekend and every Wednesday night, which allowed me to work full-time and, more importantly to me at the time, integrate my lessons into my everyday life. As so it began. Actually, I should mention that about a month before I took that course, I had taken a kids yoga training. I had no idea why; I didn't have kids or a huge affinity for them to be totally honest, but I took the course. Who knew that for the next ten years Child's Pose Yoga would be a huge part of my service and offerings, and that to hear a child tell me how her life had changed because of yoga would make my heart melt and my eyes water.

During those six months of training I learned a tremendous amount about myself and my Self. It was no small or insignificant experience. In fact, I would say it was a pivotal decision, and I feel grateful every day for having made it. The most beautiful thing about yoga is that once you have it, you have it for life. It never leaves you. You can't unknow things, and once you experience the freedom that comes from this practice, physically, mentally, emotionally, and spiritually, all you need is to access it any time you choose. It blows my mind even typing that out. Yoga can include headstands, sure, but what it meant for me was liberation—liberation from mental suffering. This is yoga. Here's the deal, as the yogis say, "Yoga is managing the fluctuations of the mind." Another lovely interpretation is "We become whole when the minds stops churning." So simple, hey? In theory, yes it is. Simple yet not necessarily easy. But as they also say, "Practice and all is coming." It isn't so much whether we master this, because let's face it, that's ambitious, since our minds are constantly jumping. But when we practice, we learn to remove some of the intensity around our thoughts and emotions. The jumping settles. If we can train our mind and show it who's boss, well then, we're on our way. As I said earlier, if we don't manage our minds, our minds will manage us. Simple. So without getting into a mini YTT of my own, there are several "paths" of yoga. I'm not talking "styles." Styles are the Western ways of compartmentalizing something so that our linear minds can understand. Yoga is yoga.

1. When I say *paths*, I'm referring to the various traditions through which one chooses to express his or her yoga:
2. devotional chant
3. self-study
4. the eight limbs, which is in a sense a guide of living a yogic lifestyle including meditation, postures, and a code of ethics if you will
5. karma yoga or selfless service, among a few others.
6. When we bring our attention and intention, and awareness of our breath to what we are doing—anytime, anywhere, anyhow—in a sense anything and everything can be yoga. For this book's purpose, I'm mentioning yoga here because it is a practice I believe in so fully and completely, and yes, it is a way to move our bodies. We learn to move calmly, steadily, intentionally, and peacefully, while also giving the mind a chance to experience the same. There is no other practice like it where embedded into each aspect of it are the underlying principles of meditation, kindness, discovery, compassion, and humility.

What I love in particular about the sun salutation series, a sequence of specifically linked postures, is that it is a moving meditation, so it does many things at once. It calms the mind, moves the body, requires some strength, feels amazing, makes me feel supple, and when practiced with some dynamic rigor, fulfills my need to increase my heart rate. When I want to relax, I simply practice it more slowly. It is a way to get in touch with your deepest self, which as you now know, is where your Inner Wild lives.

REAL LIFE EXPERIENCE

During some of the most challenging times in my life, when I thought I was losing my mind, in amidst countless anxiety attacks, some of which even brought me to the emergency room, during my separation, and when no amount of sitting to quiet my mind, or running, or wine, or talking with a friend helped, I turned to my sun salutation. It was the only thing that took me out of my head and into my body. It was the one thing that reminded me that the only thing that is real is the moment we are in, and it's hard to focus on your drama or pain when you're focusing on breathing—like really focusing on it. The mind likes to do one thing at a time. Moving through the meditation that is surya namaskar (sun salutation) is a blessing and a gift and one that keeps on giving and gets better with time. Once you practice it enough you no longer need to remember what comes next and you just go. The cool thing now is that before turning to a friend or even my journal, I turn to yoga, and it always delivers.

RECAP

—

Move at least once a day in a way that gets blood pumping and circulation moving. Yoga offers both a simple and practical experience and works on all aspects of our being. Cultivating peace while expanding our physical, emotional, and spiritual capacities is truly a remarkable thing. Yoga does not have to cost more than an intro class or a DVD to practice at home. If that doesn't suit you, simply start moving your body with care and ease, and pay attention to your breath. That is yoga. No fancy yoga pants, mats, bags, or modern-day accessories are required. What is far more important is consistency, an open heart, and the desire to learn.

Some dynamic movement is all we need to massage our hearts, flush out negative energy, and keep our bodies well oiled. A mental practice to develop mindfulness, equanimity, and joy is such a gift, and I'd argue that nothing does this more effectively or efficiently than yoga. With a new expansiveness in both the body and mind, we start to become clearer. There is more oxygen moving to and from the organs, including the brain, of course, which results in new thinking, clarity, and awareness. This is when we begin to experience our yoga—off the mat.

The best yoga advice I can give is to seek opportunities to find sweetness in your movement and in your breath; they are there just waiting to be discovered.

BE CLEAR, HAVE CLEAR BOUNDARIES, AND KNOW YOUR WORTH

This isn't a yoga book, but those yoga dudes know a thing or two, and remember, I am after all a subscriber to the practice. I am not hard-core anything, but the brilliance of yoga and all of its ancient wisdom is undeniable.

Remember those koshas, or layers, I mentioned earlier? Well, we may not always realize it, but we experience these layers frequently.

When our breath changes due to rigorous activity or from being startled, for example, we feel it. When our feelings are hurt or we experience loss or heartache, we feel that in a deep place. When our intuition kicks in, we know it. We just do. We certainly feel it in our physical bodies when a boundary has been bumped, or worse, violated. So when one or more of these other energetic layers is invaded or permeated, we will feel it too. We can't always put our finger on what the feeling is—we just get the feeling. When push comes to shove and we need to exercise these boundaries firmly, we will know how. Sometimes the only one who needs to know and understand our boundaries is us. They are like our code of conduct, a place from which we operate to ensure that our well-being and safety are protected physically, emotionally, and spiritually. And like everything I share in this book, the more we practice, the better at it we become.

If we aren't clear around our personal boundaries, things can get tricky, uncomfortable, and even downright dangerous. I've been in a situation or twenty in my life where I wish I had been clearer—both in business and in social situations. I always know what I mean; the issue is that others don't always know, so they make up their own version and take action according to *their* needs. So, it is our job to be clear.

When I am clear, I find it actually feels good because there is no deliberation or anxiety about whether I've been misunderstood. People don't always care for the boundaries I set, but that is OK. I am responsible for me. As are you for you.

A general rule in my life is "don't put someone else's feelings or well-being in front of my own." Not out of selfishness—I can be very generous. But here's the thing: if my safety or well-being is not taken care of or, worse, is at risk, I simply cannot worry about how my choices are going to offend someone. This isn't selfish—it is self-preservation, and I do it with as much compassion and kindness as I can. As I started to discover that what people think is not my responsibility, I was able to release that burden. I learned that the only responsibility I have is to me.

Back to the koshas. Be aware of when they are being poked. Notice if they are being tested; notice not so much from a cerebral place but from a feeling. If you are finding they are being prodded, it is most likely time to speak up.

For a chunk of my life when I was younger, I worried about what people thought of me, my actions, and my choices. I've even been caught up in this BS as recently as a few years ago because I allowed myself to be influenced, and I'd say disrespected by people with whom I was not meant to align, but I wasn't listening to my Spirit or higher power. It's OK. It happens. I think to a degree it is human nature to care or worry or be impressionable. It's when we dwell here that we run into trouble, remember? Examples: I have let people walk all over me because I was too afraid to speak up. I have agreed to things that didn't feel right or in line with my values because I didn't want to cause a scene. I have eaten things that were not good for me so I wouldn't offend a host. How many times have you done that!? These may seem like minor examples, but these "minor" experiences make up our lives. So, how are you showing up? How you show up in response to small boundary violations could very well be how you show up in response to the biggies.

I learned that once you waver on where the boundaries lie, it is challenging and frankly a pain in the ass to go back and reset them. It is much easier to be firm the first time around; out of our comfort zone perhaps, but it saves us effort and awkwardness later. Over time I grew clearer and clearer, experiencing a few hiccups along the way sure, but overall, I have absolutely no doubt where my boundaries lie now.

When we know who we are—in, out, and all around—we become very comfortable exercising boundaries in order to protect that. We are tested all the time by people, situations, you name it, that will quite frankly force us to stay true to our values and limits. Sometimes these boundaries are pushed, and that can cause us to re-evaluate them i.e. get clear on whether we need a boundary to be as rigid as it is and perhaps loosen it, or stick with it because it felt invasive when it was crossed.

Speak and stand up for yourself. Doing this doesn't mean you don't love someone or something, or want that someone or something in your life, but it may mean it is time to adjust, or eliminate something or someone, because you've chosen to love yourself more.

There are ("negative") things I have experienced in this lifetime that, looking back, I didn't think I deserved. But at the same time, if I was willing to put myself in that predicament and situation perhaps I did. It is not about blame or self judgment. It is simply about recognizing that we are the only ones who can take responsibility for our own wellbeing. When we take a look around and see what we're experiencing on a daily basis, we must ask if these are things we deserve. If our experiences bring feelings of joy, happiness, contentment, empowerment, and inspiration, I would say then yes, we definitely deserve them for putting ourselves in situations with positive people and high vibrations. If we are continually experiencing dread, misery, frustration, or sadness, I'm not suggesting we "deserve" those things, but it is a reminder to take a good honest look at how we're ending up in situations that create these experiences, possibly even on a repeated basis. When we start to love ourselves enough, we will start to experience these situations less and less, and then never and never. What I love about life is the opportunity to notice and without judgment make change. I love how people come into my life for various reasons, and how it is *my* job to decide what to do with my energy and its direction as it relates to said people. I always have my own back, because I trust myself to know what is best for me. On the occasion where I find myself in a situation that doesn't feel good, I examine why and then I change my trajectory toward something that does. Either way, I am responsible for me, and I am the only one who puts myself into situations. There is nothing more empowering than knowing your worth and then not accepting anything less than what you deserve. This way there is no blame, only accountability.

RECAP

The more we know ourselves and what is important to us, our value systems, and our non-negotiables, the clearer our boundaries become, and the more we will do whatever it takes to honour them.

SPEAK YOUR TRUTH

There is a word in Sanskrit—satya—which translates to truth. In the context of yoga, we are taught to be honest. Similar to "thou shalt not lie," but instead of a demand or a big, bad voice pointing a finger at you with a threat, it is framed in the positive—be honest.

In theory, this is great—let's all be honest and the world will be a better place.

In my experience, when people are honest there can be a lack of awareness around *how* this honesty is being shared. People don't always realize how their honesty comes through, or they are so busy self-proclaiming as "straight shooters" or someone with "no filter" that the respect and mindfulness aspect of the honesty is nowhere to be found or heard. Be honest, speak truthfully, totally. Here's the caveat: according to yogic wisdom and simply "just" being a good human, use discretion in your honesty.

Is yours a truth that *needs* to be spoken, or is your ego just dying to get in there and give your opinion?

Pause. Reflect. Notice. Can what you are saying with honesty be said with love for all, in a non-harming way (ahimsa, the preceding "code of ethics" just before satya), or will it cause another person so much pain that perhaps it is better left unsaid? Only you know, case by case. When we come from a place of non-harming, we can express and articulate our truths in the interest of wanting to support this other human on his or her path to wholeness, *not* from a place of anger, resentment, hostility, ego, or frustration. If you did a little check-in with your emotions and had this person's best interest at heart as well as your need for getting something off your chest or proving a point or being right, how might you re-frame your truth? Whether this person is a loved one or the server at a restaurant who has provided poor service. Pause. Reflect. Notice.

Hey, I get it, sometimes you just wanna be like "Look here _____(appropriate expletive) blah blah blah blah." When we frame our truth this way (direct, accusatory, etc.), it often falls on deaf ears anyway, because the host environment is not one of hearing or receiving. Can you blame the other person? And not to say we are always lashy-outty, but in the heat of a share, things can escalate quickly. It is likely that our emotional sheath has been poked. Going into a conversation with intention for both or all people's highest good sets the stage for a peaceful exchange. It may require continuous revisits even during that one conversation, depending on how it goes. I often have to remind myself of my intention: honouring my truth while honouring the other person as well. Annoying, I know, but this is our job as conscious humans. It definitely requires continuous practice, and I am not always great at it either, but I make conscious efforts to be. When I'm not, I examine what I could have done differently and what I can do next time to create a more positive outcome.

> Question—When was a time you recently shared your truth in a way that resulted in feelings being hurt and things being spoken that you now wish you could take back? *Or* when was the last time you wanted to share a truth but didn't feel equipped, so you just didn't and now it's sitting in your gut, liver, or throat? What do you need to do in order to release this truth in a respectful, high-frequency way so that it doesn't fester and suppress your Inner Wild that is making valiant efforts to emerge?

The more we can speak the truth from a place of compassion and strength, the more we can be role models for others on how to live their truth authentically. Remember, Wild does't mean gruff, aggressive or intimidating. It means being connected to Spirit, yours and the Spirits of those around you. It means being harmonious with our environment. When someone has a positive exchange with you due to your emotional intelligence and your kind, respectful expression of your truth, they may walk away surprised and even inspired to try it for themselves. Then what we have are more people in the world sharing conscious awareness-communication, rather than having a bunch of loose cannons, or carriers of unspoken truths walking around. You can be a part of creating this shift. Do it.

Learning to use my voice was a scary thing. As a teen I was often the first person to mouth off or be sassy. But when it came time to choose and use my words kindly, slowly, and to honour myself and my needs, I would become small. I would think *What if I lose this person?* or *What if they get mad and it becomes a whole big thing?* Well, guess what. Both of those things happened either way, and more often as a result of me bottling up feelings and then a month or year later erupting like a fricken volcano. So, over time, I became clearer about how certain situations or behaviours or vibrations made me feel. Yes, I could go on about how nothing or no one makes us feel anything without our permission, blah blah blah, but the truth is when we are in tune with ourselves, we notice when certain situations create a positive, healthy vibe, and when others don't. Using my voice became easier, not because I suddenly decided to "speak up," but because I gradually, with practice, started to honour myself more. It was like my spirit wouldn't stay quiet any longer. The beautiful thing is that through my yoga practice, I learned how to use my voice in a way that is kinder. With more practice, it became easier, or at least less horrifying. It didn't always work out perfectly. If the other person was offended or upset or chose to leave as a result, I needed to be OK with that. In time, that became easier too.

Sometimes speaking our truth can be a one-off situational thing. Other times it is bigger than that. When we live life according to a relationship, a job, or anything else that is not directed by our own intelligence—the intuitive third-eye intelligence—then we are living according to someone else's truth, their rules, or limitations, and ultimately we lose ourselves. For those who are in a partnership, it can be tricky for sure to live in union with someone and remain true to yourself. I believe this is why people have affairs or stay in unhappy marriages, or change jobs every two years in search of a "better", more fulfilling one. People lose themselves because they don't know who they really are, and once they discover this, they don't know how to communicate it in a kind, respectful, and truthful way. So they blame their partner, their kids, their boss. This is where we can get into trouble. Over time, resentments build and one day we erupt. Things are said that can't be retracted. And on it goes. We have all been there, on both ends. Both kinda suck.

Once again, we need to get very clear on who we are, what our truth is, and what are the non-negotiables. Then life becomes less complicated, because there are things we are no longer willing to accept … and then a really cool thing starts to happen. High vibes start comin' and the rest falls away. It's pure magic. Self-made magic.

Picking up on a general theme yet? Know Thyself. The practices in this book will help you get there. I will go so far as to say these practices will save you. Keep working your way toward your Inner Wild. She is waiting for you.

RECAP

—

Before you speak your truth, consider if what you are sharing needs to be spoken.
If it does, how can you do it in a way that honours both you and the recipient of your truth?
When you do this, two things happen: First, your confidence develops,
and it becomes easier to make this part of who you are. The second thing that
happens is that people come to expect it from you, and because your truths
come with respect and love, they are actually received.

HAVE CONFIDENCE, TRUST YOUR GUT, AND TAKE RISKS

Generally speaking, I believe that we do our best with what we have at the time. There have been times however where I could have done better, and not just in hindsight. Times when I felt something "off" and chose not to follow my gut. I won't call these mistakes, only lessons or reminders of what I already knew, but I *will* say I have a new respect for my gut. It has literally never led me astray. The times I felt betrayed by my gut I examined the situations more closely and realized that it was in fact doing its job, I simply didn't listen. Most of the time though, I do. Here are some examples:

I can say that in the last fifteen years I have taken some major life risks. As recently as two years ago, when I moved to this town to start a new business, I basically started life over at forty-three, and I *knew* in my deepest place that I was going to be OK. I really mean that. How did I know? I just did. When we take a risk, a major one, and we see that we are OK or perhaps even better than before in a way, it builds our belief in the not yet seen. It gives us the strength and courage to keep taking risks.

What I learned from taking big risks is that the Universe catches us. See, the Universe is us, and we are the Universe and it responds back with whatever we put out there. So we don't have to thank the Universe for anything; we can thank ourselves for being bold. Our willingness to risk and jump is rewarded, because we will be caught by Community, in a hammock of grace, or in something with more bounce, and in ways we can never imagine until we are bold and blessed enough to experience them.

When I do what is best for my highest Self, scary or not, when I come from a place of being in service to others, doing what will give me the greatest opportunity to share my gifts, even if that means saying goodbye to people, places, or things, I know I will land on my feet, or in a hammock, or bouncy castle. Over time, my faith in this notion of being rewarded, or caught, or whatever we want to call it— not left to just hit a pile of rocks—is unwavering. Each time I take a risk and land safely, it affirms for me that risk, when taken with intelligence, highest good, and our best interest at heart, is rewarded. Magnificently.

REAL LIFE EXPERIENCE

In December of 2001, I got engaged. A year and a half earlier, I had met the fellow who would become my fiancé, when my sister asked me to co-MC her wedding. He was the co. We met, and I wouldn't say there was a "spark," but apparently something led me to get engaged. I was twenty-eight years old, and it was all good. Real convincing huh? Fast forward from her wedding, to his proposal—I remember feeling somewhat sick when I was given this most incredible solitaire, square diamond. This gem was as clear as Caribbean waters and was "totally me", whatever that means. Only one thing was wrong: I knew it wasn't me. I mean, the diamond may have been my style, but it wasn't the right situation. I thought at first it was just the butterflies you hear about. Nerves. The kind that make you want to super puke. I went ahead and started planning the wedding for October 2002. Frankly, nothing about it felt right, not even the date—it was going to be on October thirteenth. *Oy* is right. I enjoyed trying on gowns, I won't lie, and I bought a gorgeous mocha-coloured, two-piece gown fit for a princess. Actually, it was more like caramel, but not important.

Fast forward many months, and my anxiety worsened. I actually experienced my first severe anxiety attack. Not only was I becoming more and more certain this was the wrong person for me, but I'd met someone in those months who I quickly realized was the *right* person. Double *oy*. I had the right kind of butterflies, the schoolgirl kind of giddiness every time I saw him, which was daily because he worked one floor above me. Triple *oy*. I even recall saying to him "is it hot in here or is it just me" one morning when we bumped into each other, although I am sure I had no actual business on his floor at 7am that day. So yeah, I was in all sorts of trouble. Still avoiding what I knew was true and undeniable, fiancé and I left Vancouver, where we were living at the time, and of course where "Mr. Right" lived, and we headed east to rural Ontario, in a car might I add, where we were planning to start our new life. *Oy oy oy oy*. I had spoken to many people prior to my departure to express my fears and feelings. "It's normal," said one person. "Every bride goes through this," said another. And so I continued. We drove as far as Winnipeg, where we stopped in to see my parents. This was the beginning of the end and the end of the beginning. Each day that we were there, which was four in total, I think, I'd check the mailbox only to see RSVPs piling up. With each check I'd feel more and more sick. It was four weeks away. Everything was done. Deposits were paid. Many flights were booked. Gifts were opened and thank-you cards sent. I'll skip some details but basically that was it. This was where the wedding was called off, the ring returned, and where I experienced Jewish guilt like no other. I'd wasted my parents' money. I ruined someone's life. OMG.

A day or so later as he left to carry on to Ontario, solo, I decide to jump in as he pulled out of the driveway. Actually. Literally, he was backing out. I asked him to wait five minutes while I tossed a bag together and made a call to Vancouver and explained that I needed to complete this journey but that I'd be back. Mr. Right was very understanding. And for the record, there was no affair, just a feeling in my heart that I knew he was the one.

I continued on to Ontario to "help" with the drive and get closure, or whatever I called it, in order to see this thing to the end and then let it go. I stayed in Toronto for a month or two with my sis before heading back to Vancouver. People thought I was nuts. Risk #2—Going back to a city where I had no job, not many friends, no money, and nothing more than that hockey bag with my then-possessions and I believe a broken zipper. Yes, I gave up my furniture, returned the wedding gifts and $, and carried on. I tell you this why? Because it is the clearest example of how I trusted my gut. Not once but twice. Two big risks in a short period of time, both of which changed the trajectory of my life in the most major of ways. First, I listened to my intuition—in fact, I had no other choice. I simply could not go through with it, out of respect for everyone. I knew that despite causing a lot of pain, I was doing the right thing. 1000000%.

Then I followed my gut again and what do ya know, Mr. Right and I lived in partnership for the next fourteen years. What a gift. We know what we know. We can be told this, that, and the other. It don't make a damn bit of difference when we know what we know, when we feel what we feel. There is a reason it is called our gut feeling. Feel it. Listen to it. It won't steer you wrong.

Now that you're all confident, you can

LET GO & FREE YOURSELF.
IF YOU WANT TO BE WILD, YOU NEED TO MASTER THIS

Whether or not you choose to adore or listen to the Buddha, I think it is fair to say he had it goin' on; he had some pretty clever insights into human suffering and also into liberation. According to Buddha and his discoveries as he set out into the world to understand the cause of human suffering, attachment is in fact the cause. Let's look at this more closely.

Buddha taught these Four Noble Truths:

1) All existence is suffering. 2) Suffering comes from grasping, or pushing (i.e. wanting something to be different than it is). 3) The way to cessation of suffering is non-grasping. 4) There is an eight-fold path that can take us there.

Let's examine grasping:

Have you ever noticed that when you hold onto something, eventually your hand starts to hurt? When we grip something, someone, an idea, or even an emotion, ultimately we suffer. Holding on to people, thoughts, situations, experiences, emotions, or relationships doesn't make them ours, and it certainly doesn't increase the chances of having them forever. In fact, it is likely that the tighter we squeeze, the more pain we will cause and in turn the more likely we will lose said person, thing, or idea. Because the thing is, nothing is ours to hold. Not. A. Thing.

We can choose to enjoy life while we are here. We can choose to love fully and love up on our people and give our relationships our all. We can even "love" our new car or condo, as long as we also understand that nothing is ours and nothing is forever.

We have a limited time on earth, so we can either live the hell out of it all-in, or we can hold back and not love fully out of fear we will get hurt or lose something—meaning if we live out of fear, we often attach to someone far beyond what is reasonable, and in the end we lose them anyway. But let's not confuse grasping with loving fully.

Now, we can choose to see this impermanence as something to grieve or something to celebrate. The choice is ours and, as always, it is important to remember this.

Even in the most seemingly unbearable times and situations, we have the choice to let go, and by that I mean let go of the desperate desire to stop suffering. Sometimes our desire and our hold isn't even on a person or relationship, but rather it is a deep desire to want to not feel what we are feeling. Letting go works in two ways: letting go of attachment to people, things, and experiences, and letting go of our desire to need things to be different. Sometimes this means we need to suffer and be sad and grieve and let go of our desire for it to pass. Make sense?

Some people will choose to dwell in sadness or grief, hardship or pain, and others will seem to "handle" or process it more easily. I can promise you it isn't because it is easier. Day after day, sometimes even moment to moment, those people are choosing consciously to make their experience a more pleasant, love-filled one than one of pain and suffering. They are doing the work.

It is possible that some people are hard-wired genetically to be happier, more positive, or more optimistic, but it is definitely something that can be learned and practiced and even mastered over time. Some will choose to ignore the pain by way of denial or distraction. This might come in the form of substance misuse or abuse, by projecting anger or fear or finding a way to blame others for their situation and currently reality. Some will sit with it until it lessens over time. I can say from experience that the latter isn't easy, but it is the only real way.

ON ATTACHMENT

Material things like a house, a car, or a new cutting edge device are often disguised as happiness. Money, money, money is often what people believe will bring happiness, but at the root, all we truly want and need is actual happiness, inner peace, and contentment … or what yogis call santosha. Yes, again with the yoga, but it's made sense so far, right?

We've seen it in Hollywood and in our own lives—people who seem to have "everything" may still be depressed, disengaged, or suicidal, yet we still believe that material wealth is the answer. People still chase the money. Why??!? Because they haven't done the inner work. They don't want to sit with themselves in a quiet place, and these material things offer a distraction so that they don't have to. I may upset some readers by saying this but hell, some people keep having kids and more kids, not even aware that this too can be a distraction! Things, people, and experiences bring temporary pleasure. No doubt. From chocolate to vacations to cars to shiny diamonds or new bohemian sandals, you name it. And hey, there is nothing wrong with enjoying these things. I love me some good chocolate and a trip to Hawaii. It is our attachments to and the significance we give these things that cause us pain. Why? Because they are temporary. They break, get lost, or end, and then we have to deal with losing them, and so we suffer. We aren't taught as kids that everything in life is temporary, including life. I mean, we all know people die, but we aren't taught how to accept the end of things. We just aren't.

We aren't given the skills to process loss, and so we suffer, immensely, and then we want more things to replace the things we've lost. It is a never-ending cycle.

When we are content inside, in our innermost place, it makes less of a difference whether these things come or go. We can still enjoy them fully and completely, and then we can release them.

Nothing is permanent. Not the things or not having the things. It all comes and goes, and when we are truly centered, none of it matters.

When we cultivate happiness inside by detaching from people, things, and even our emotions, we can sit back as witnesses to these people, things, and emotions as they come and go, without attaching to them. We experience them as fully as we can and then release them. This doesn't mean we won't experience deep loss, sadness, grief, and other significant emotions. It means we learn to become witnesses to those emotions rather than becoming them. Yes this repeated a bit but I think it is worth repeating and I am not sure if you'll go back and re-read (wink).

It took me forty-five years to fully get this. Not just intellectually, but *get it* in my cells and bones.

I had called off a wedding and started life over with the man of my dreams. I was pretty sure I'd just learned a hard lesson in letting go and felt I had earned the right to enjoy the fruits of my decision making and bravery for a long time to come, maybe forever. Riiiiight, but nothing lasts forever. Oh the irony. Little did I know that in order to reap the benefits of honouring one's Wild, one has to stay true to that Wild and always, always pay attention. I had no idea that yet another lesson in letting go, an even harder one, would eventually come my way again. For thirteen years, Mr. Right and I went on vacations, lived in some pretty amazing homes, moved into a condo we couldn't really afford, but it had a hot tub, pool, sauna, steam room, gym, *and* a concierge! We had so much fun, and the real kind, swankiness stuff aside—we laughed a ton. Life was good. I was sure this was the way the rest of my adult years would be spent. I solidified my dream job on a regular term, not just a contract, and I got a raise—life was grand in fact.

I had a great job, a gorgeous boat, a beautiful home, a wonderful partner... all of these added up to a pretty sweet life. It probably even looked enviable to those looking in. We had it all. Or did we?

I had it all until I realized that I didn't. Fast forward some time and now something wasn't totally right. I wasn't feeling whole. I realize now that I unfairly expected my partner to make me feel whole. Of course, now I know wholeness comes from a deep, inner, spiritual place, but at the time, even though I thought I understood this, I was still searching for something, and none of these things, not even my newfound love of yoga teaching, could fill me up. Why? Because they were outside of me. And so I knew this meant I needed to pursue a deep investigation. I learned the hard way that anything outside of me was not inside of me. And anything not inside of me was outside of me. Seems obvious, hey? Not exactly. We know this intellectually, yet we still grasp at external, material things to fill us. I was still hoping something would fill the gap, but I also knew that wouldn't work long term. I had my work cut out for me, and I was dreading it, quite honestly.

It was like I knew in my gut with each day that passed that there was this mountain I needed to climb, but I didn't have the right gear, training, and/or desire to embark on this journey. I wanted my life as I knew it to be perfect as it was. I'd worked damn hard to get there. I'd taken risks. Spoken my truth. I'd earned the right for this to work and last forever! I didn't want it to change.

It was a very painful lesson when I realized it had, when I awoke to it. I knew I needed to live a different life, one that didn't remotely resemble my current one.

When that reality set in, my heart broke into what felt like a billion pieces. Maybe more. It stayed broken for a long time. Years in fact. Sometimes I still cry.

One day in December of 2014, it was like a lightbulb flashed—literally. My partner and I both knew that our time together was coming to an end. In fact, it was probably overdue, and not because there was a lack of love; in fact, it was quite the opposite. There was so much love that we wanted the other to be happy and free, and we recognized we were better people apart than we were together. We decided in what seemed like overnight to sell our home and amicably go our separate ways. How absolutely heartbreaking. We both deserved to be happy and we knew that happiness looked different for each of us. It wasn't one or the other. It was just time and as heartbroken as we both were, we knew it was what needed to happen. But after all we had been through, and the fairytale it had been, or seemed, I was still in disbelief.

In an attempt to step outside of my situation and clear my head, better known as an escape, I went down to Mexico for ten days to see my folks. I figured some space, time, and family connection would help me look at this surreal situation with new eyes. At the end of that trip, I came back to Vancouver and decided to request some unpaid time off from my job at the university. Yes, it was a risk. I woke up that day and was prepared to ask for three months off, unsure of where I would live, what I would do for money, or really, what the hell I was going to do in general, but I knew I needed that time to devote to my healing. I attended a meeting to make my request, and before I had even opened my mouth to make said request, I was told my position had been eliminated while I was away. I would no longer be working for the university effective that moment. I would receive a severance and was to clear out my desk and basically be gone, in an hour. Well, that was a bit of a shocker. What in the actual …had just happened?

So within a three-week period, a separation from my partner, job of thirteen years eliminated, selling of my home … here I was, experiencing loss and anxiety on levels I had never known, and all at once. At least knowing I had some financial support helped to keep me from panicking on that front. But letting go of things I thought I'd have "forever," or at least a very long time, was a very painful thing to endure.

I had to let go of my home and everything that living in Vancouver represented. In essence, I was saying goodbye to all of the things that brought me feelings of safety and security. I kind of felt like the ground had been pulled out from under me. I had to let go of the deep connections and then, yes, the less-important stuff like the comforts that money and all the organic juice bars and yoga studios within walking distance can bring. Perhaps these things seem unimportant, but these were my life's moments, my daily ways of being. It took "losing" everything, in a sense, to gain other things, which, granted, came years later. Things like peace of mind and ease of heart, and a different kind of happiness. I released material things, attachment to human relationships, and my thoughts and beliefs on how some things were supposed to go. All of it.

So I had two choices: dwell or deal. I was now on my own essentially, so dwelling wasn't a practical option. That said, I think it's OK to dwell for a bit. We all need our moments where we cry, have a pity party, and ask *why me, how did this happen, when did this happen, now what?* Do what you need to do to let it all out and then make a conscious decision not to dwell here.

I believe, looking back, that I was drifting through this experience at times. It was indeed surreal. We have all heard the expression "brought me to my knees." Well, this experience did that for me, and it was humbling to say the least. It was the time when I learned that the only way back to peace was to turn in.

I also had enough sense, however, to keep putting one foot in front of the other until I reached safety. It took time—moving through the stages of loss. I went on a journey of self-discovery. I had some less than pretty experiences along the way. I had moments where I didn't even know who I was, and while I was able to witness that at times from outside of myself, I was not quite able to gently coach myself back to centre. I allowed the actions of others to greatly impact my feeling of self-worth and self-esteem. I lost sight of my values, and in hindsight I see now that I was in survival mode. And then, then I emerged. Bit by bit I regained my voice, only this time I had developed a sense of grace that wasn't there before. I evolved into someone stronger and more sure than ever, of who I am. I realized I was actually in this alone and I only had me to count on. I had friends and family sure, but at the end of the day I was responsible for my situation, where I'd live, how I'd get there, how I'd earn an income all over again, and ultimately for how I felt. I was responsible for my life. Me. No one else. I needed to get to work.

What I also realized, of course, was that I had always been responsible for these things, but having a partner lessens the load, and at times muddies these waters, tricking us into thinking "this" is someone else's work. It isn't.

So as I began to wake from the fog, I discovered a new person inside … well, more like an improved version of the already fabulous me, and one who would now choose herself first, from this point forward. No blaming or accusations or judgment, but a definite shift in how I viewed the world, love, and life.

I let go of many things that year: pieces of me, a lot of pain, suffering, confusion, and expectations. In my heart I let go of a love I thought was invincible. There are moments even to this day that I can't believe it but this doesn't mean it didn't happen exactly as it needed to. It all brought me to this moment. I look at love and loss in an entirely new way. I hold dear each experience for the gifts it offers *now*. I remind myself that nothing is forever, and this has allowed me to invite in an appreciation of the present that I hadn't understood or experienced before. The love I experience now is different and without expectation, and this is a remarkable gift in itself. To love without attachment is really extraordinary. All of this took a great deal of introspection and self-examining. How wonderful to be able to say I came through and here I am stronger than ever and more certain that I am always OK. Always. And so are you. Right now.

GET REAL

What do you need to let go of? How can you ensure you are supported fully and completely as you shed what you need to and open up to new possibilities and ways of life?

What are you attached to? Why are you attached?

Yes, this may be a place where you wanna hurt me a bit, or cry, or scream. DO IT! Well, not the hurt me part.

Get clear with yourself; get real with yourself.

RECAP

Letting go of things, ideas, emotions, or relationships creates space for new things to move in. So often we miss out on the brilliance of life because we are holding on to the past or an idea of what the future should look like. We can miss out on things that can raise our vibe and bring us closer to our life's purpose. Everything is a stepping stone to greatness. We simply need to pay attention and notice and respect when it is time to step. When we do, a sense of ease and peace washes over us. I promise. And your Inner Wild takes yet one more step forward.

Side bar: I wanted to write a book on amicable separations. Here we were, two people who'd thought we'd live to 100 and then turn to stardust together, and instead we found ourselves saying goodbye, knowing we were better people individually than we were together. What a lesson in what it means to love, and to let go. I am delighted to say we are still the greatest of friends. Never once did I consider the end of that relationship as it was, a failure or something that didn't work. It worked until it didn't, and it is something that I celebrate … all stages and aspects of it. If we even need to use the word, *failure* would be not having changed a situation that wasn't bringing out the best in two people. Let's start celebrating people who make hard choices; frig, let's start a (sustainable) greeting card line that says *"Congratulations on your separation! You are strong and bold and supported—way to go for taking care of your heart and soul and for freeing up another's!"*

Remember:

What we want in life, we can create, whether that is a dream job, a certain lifestyle, or staying friends with an ex-partner.

PLEASURES

One of my favourite lines of all time that I read not too long ago said "I do a thing called what I want." So let me take that one step further and say I stay Wild by doing a thing called what I want.

When you let go … you have more space to enjoy. It may take time, but it will come.

This is hard for many. It has been my experience that it is more often women who struggle with this, whether it is because they have taken on the notion that they shouldn't enjoy, or that it's selfish, or they simply don't know how.

I am happy to report I am not one of those women. In fact, I am a master of enjoying pleasures, which is why I feel I can speak on the subject. I never really struggled with this, but there was a stage in my life where I spent too much time not doing the "things called what I want," so now I'm making up for lost time. Every single day I do what I want. Literally. *And* I stopped doing things I don't want to do. Period. These are two different things. It's "double trouble," and by trouble I mean awesomeness.

I may not have kids and a million responsibilities associated with that, but even when I worked nine to five, was running a biz, taking yoga training, and engaging in other activities that required my energy, I *always* made sure I carved out Dana time. I reaped the benefit and in turn so did my students, friends, relationships, and my work. It isn't about putting oneself "first," because people get hung up on that and whether it is selfish, and then it gets all martyr-y. I mean I put myself first but I don't think it is selfish. Simply put, it is essential to your well-being to take time to feel your feet on the ground and your head on your shoulders, and to have your mind at least somewhat in order. So don't think for one second that because you have kids or a full-time job or aging parents or all of it that you can't enjoy simple pleasures. You can. *Now,* not in ten years.

It may require more effort and coordination, but it's doable. Now, before you get all poopy with me and tell me I don't get it because I don't have kids—it's true, I don't, but I have spent lots of time with parents. I teach a lot of moms with toddlers, and I see and honour their commitment to their wellness, not to mention their sanity. It is possible. There are ways.

Whether you're a mom, a dad, a single parent, or someone who feels you don't have time to create the life you want, here is a newsflash … You are the only one who can make the choices that will shape your life.

Let's read that again. You are the *only* one who can make the choices that will shape your life.

If you aren't doing what you want, my suggestion is to get real clear on why that is and then examine that even further. Is it easier to complain than to actually make stuff happen? Just asking.

Doing what you want doesn't have to mean taking a two-month trip to Fiji, because perhaps that is simply not practical given your job, family, financial, or time resources. That doesn't mean you can't do something you want to do at least once a day. Choose it and then I strongly advise you to write it down on your list of things to do and do it. Take back the power that is yours to create the life you want to live. Choice by choice by choice.

Next thing you know, you're no longer doing things you don't want to do and you've replaced those with things you WANT to do.

There are lots of things you can do that will bring you small pleasures that also remind you that your life is now and you deserve and need to start enjoying it. Extremely.

Pause here and now and write down one thing you can enjoy, extremely, today, that won't require you to save money, request time off, get permission, or make any elaborate plans.

Eat the chocolate, have the espresso, take that pole fit class … wait, those are my things. But in all seriousness, do something you enjoy, something that brings you pleasure in tiny amounts, or large, or better yet, both.

I decide when I wake up what I will do, how I will enjoy my morning … and that is a gift I am very much aware of. A gift that I choose to give myself in this life, each day.

If you need to wake up five minutes before the rest of your household in order to get these small but *significant* moments of pleasure in, then do it. If you choose to stay in bed that's also a pleasure. Whatever it is that you choose, choose it, own it, and love up on it. Do what brings you pleasure, and the more you do it, the more it becomes a habit. If having time to yourself each morning is important to you, you'll find the five bonus minutes, I promise you.

RECAP

——

Whatever your pleasures are, enjoy them! Fully. Extremely.

FUEL YOUR WILD SELF

Becoming a strong, confident, Wild, high-vibe spiritual badass means having somewhere for that energy to live and thrive.

Remember, in the wild there is order. The way we do everything matters. The food we put into our bodies is among the top, if not *the* top, priority. Remember my passion disclaimer?

It's funny, as in "funny" how the one thing we can control that has the greatest impact on our well-being and thus our ability to thrive in this lifetime in our own wild way, is the thing we compromise partly because of time but mainly because of money. Yet we find money for cigarettes, alcohol, concerts, trips, and junk food. It is not possible to reach a higher frequency when we are polluting our bodies with garbage. Sorry, truth.

Ever look at an image of vegetables, fruit, seeds, nuts, and rice bowls and then look at an image of cookies, crackers, donuts, fast food burgers, and pizza? Which one looks vital? Which one looks dormant or dead? This isn't a trick question. The answer is pretty easy. Eat food that is alive and it will give you life. Eat food that is dormant or dead, well … you will likely feel that way too. If not immediately then over time, because once the instant, happy feeling we get from sugar and chemicals found in fast food, or in "treats" like ice cream or cakes wears off, and it always does, we feel like crap. Our bodily systems are so deeply and intricately connected that when we consume low-vibration food, our emotional health is impacted as well. Sometimes we feel guilty and ashamed, frustrated, or even angry at ourselves, followed by feeling depressed, and so we turn to this food again to bring us temporary happiness or comfort. Here is where a very dangerous cycle of emotional eating often begins.

When we raise our vibrations, we build a capacity within our bodies, and we do this by way of high-vibration energy—AKA food. If we want to create and live a life that is wild, vibrant, positive, and healthy, we need to put that in us to start. Plain and simple.

We all need to eat to survive. Many of us enjoy eating and are blessed with the resources to make that happen. Some of us have more, some of us have less, but if you bought this book, it's safe to say you're doing OK and are affording some kind of food. Let's take a look at fueling our bodies, and how critical it is to our overall wellness and wildness.

We've all heard the expression "you are what you eat." This is a biggie. We may not always want to think about it, but truer words were never spoken. Our food becomes us. It becomes our muscles, our hair, teeth, and organs. What we feed our body we feed our brain, and our brain of course governs all, so it is important to take stock and ask, and get real here—what are we feeding ourselves? What are we putting into ourselves? Are we using our privilege of food as a way to heal, or harm us? This isn't a judgment. It is a question that only you can answer. My invitation, in fact, is to answer without judgment, only honesty. Start where you are. I asked myself this question year after year as I wondered why I did not feel quite at home in my body. It is something I continue to ask myself each time I am about to make food choices. If that feels like a burden to you, I get it, but rather than taking that on as a heavy thing, I view it as an honour, a freedom … I get to choose, and so I also choose to feel grateful for this opportunity to eat, an opportunity that so many people don't get.

Many of us have also at one time or another struggled with body image, weight loss or gain issues, and generally speaking have had a yin yang relationship with food. I certainly have. I went on my first diet when I was eighteen, and life with food as I knew it changed and became so complicated after that. I was 118 pounds, so yeah, didn't need to be on a diet, but I had decided I wanted to be. I dropped down to 104 pounds and within a few months and lots of binging bumped back up to 137. Good times.

I am glad to say that I no longer struggle and haven't for at least ten years.

Here is what I've come to learn, love, and believe about food. I promised you simple. Quite simply put, food has the power to heal us or harm us. Nothing novel there. I believe every choice we make about what, how, when, and why to ingest food determines whether said food will heal or harm us. Hippocrates coined the phrase, "Let food be thy medicine, and medicine be thy food." So while it may seem daunting at first, it really is simple. How do I want to feel and will this food experience contribute or take away from that feeling?

I love the way fresh, life-giving food makes me feel both physically and emotionally. Whole, nourishing food fuels and nourishes our bodies. Processed, fake, and manufactured "food" doesn't. Again, it's quite simple. This is not a judgment or opinion. It's a truth. And hey, for the record, I'm not naïve; I'm at a place on my organic, earth-giving, natural, hippie path where I am also cool to admit that not all health food always tastes amazing, but one thing is for certain and that is whole, fresh, seasonal, vibrant, alive food (in yoga known as sattvic) contributes to these same qualities once it is ingested. Stale, contaminated, preserved, highly processed "food" (in yoga known as tamasic) causes us to feel lethargic, lazy, bloated, unwell, and the opposite of vital.

Whenever possible, I choose high-vibe food, food that is alive, something that makes my cells go, "Oh yeah, baby, thank you, jump jump"—food that is not mass produced; food that uses the least amount of packaging and of course food rich in nutrients. When I can't do that, I make other choices. That's all. No judgment. No drama. Just choices. Choices I don't need to weigh or overthink or have residual feelings about. Goes something like, "In this moment, what is the best choice I can make that will contribute to my highest potential and feeling of well-being?" Sometimes that looks like a dark chocolate bar … I mean piece of dark chocolate. Other times it looks like a big, green, crunchy salad, and other times it looks like a kick-ass burger. It really depends. One thing I do is let my body guide what I eat, and in turn it takes good care of me. On the occasions where I let my mind take over, like the times I tell myself, "I deserve a treat" and proceed to have too much of something like sugar or grease, my body tells me later it isn't happy with me. Or when I ignore my desire for something, eat ten other things in an attempt to fill the gap only to come back to that desirable taste anyway and thus overeat and get cranky. This happens very infrequently now but it is an example of overthinking and moving from a place of think vs. feel. It is a beautiful thing, in fact—listening. Loving. Appreciating. Honouring. Respecting. Grounding. This is where I connect with my Inner Wild—the voice that reminds me where I want to be. What I need. That deeply intelligent guide. She never leaves. She always knows.

As a rule, I tune into my needs and I trust that my instincts will lead me down the right path.

In the wild there are a couple of options food-wise. Animal. Plants. Annnd, oh yeah, that's it. Man and woman survived on that for what … millions of years before manufactured "food" was introduced? We ate real food that grew in nature and that had life-giving qualities. Not only did it feed us, it nourished us.

Notice your relationship with food. How can you bring balance, respect, and appreciation to your eating experiences? As I said earlier, so many people don't have the privilege of experiencing food.

So how can we honour this privilege? How can we experience an exchange?

Gratitude for sustenance.

Appreciation for nourishment.

Acceptance and integration for nutrition and vitality.

Here are some very practical food habits that will leave you feeling whole, nourished, and well.

- Eat when you're hungry and don't eat when you're not. Imagine if we all did this. Emotions are so beautiful, and connecting with them is what allows us as humans to be so unique and blessed. Emotions, however, when not managed (that definition of Wild that pertains to destructive, pleasure-seeking behaviour), can be the cause of harm, at times in the form of aggressive words, behaviour, and self-inflicted pain, such as abuse of substances, including food.

- Be gentle with yourself when you've eaten the "wrong" thing. Be forgiving. If you start to fall into a pattern of emotional eating, that's OK. We've all done it. Inquire with yourself, stay curious, journal, peel it back, and see if you can resolve it. Or simply move on. Guilt, self-loathing, blame, and punishment do not deserve a seat at the dinner table, so don't invite them.

- Take a moment before "taking" or ingesting food. Someone somewhere, ideally close to home though that's not always possible, worked very hard in order for us to have this easily accessible sustenance. Giving thanks before eating can truly transform our experience. I find it slows me down similarly to how my morning gratitude practice slows me down. I often look at my food, appreciating its colours and beauty. Then I close my eyes and take in the aromas. It feels nice to appreciate my food.

- Be flexible. Obviously I am an advocate for whole, fresh, organic, seasonal, life-giving nourishment. But I am accepting and awake to the fact that life isn't always a perfect formula, and the less rigid we are, both physically and energetically, the more likely we are to experience the gifts of each moment and situation. There is something awesome and even wild about eating a street smokey while strolling the seawall on a hot summer night. We can miss these opportunities if we are totally rigid, needing organic, perfect food served and consumed in a particular way.

- Again it comes back to choice. I'm not saying eat the mini donuts, the smokey, a milkshake, and a pound of caramel corn only to feel like dying after. I'm saying be flexible and make the choices that are the best for you in each moment. Humans are known to rebel, break diets, and eat everything in sight, all under the terms "cheat day" or "balance." This isn't balance. It is harmful and abusive behaviour toward oneself. Keep your head on, make choices, and then enjoy those choices fully.

- How we eat is just as important as what we eat. If we are considering that humans are complex, multifaceted beings, we must then consider more than one aspect to the very thing that sustains us. Our beings have many layers, each one requiring something different. My offering to you as you read these pages is to invite in awareness to a holistic way of being. This doesn't mean wearing hemp pants and sitting in lotus position to eat. Holistic has become a word associated with hippies, naturalists, off-gridders, and the like. Not that there's anything wrong with any of these "types", in fact I'm a bit of each of them. Holistic, simply put, means *whole*. Interconnected. And since we are made up of many intricate systems, it only makes sense that we start treating ourselves that way. It is important to note that the energy in our food can have a drastic impact on our digestion and how our body assimilates this food. Example: an organic salad eaten under stress in a noisy environment while in a hurry or on the phone may, in fact, cause more harm than a greasy burger enjoyed on the beach with a loved one, sharing stories while feeling relaxed and content. Even if we are feeling happy and excited but rushed while we eat, this can impact our body's ability to process food. We may experience actual signs in real time, i.e. indigestion, heartburn, needing to run to the bathroom, etc... We may not experience immediate effects, but that doesn't mean they aren't taking place. How we ingest and digest our food matters. Our gut contains more neurons than that of the spinal column and peripheral nervous systems. These neurons are known as the second brain. The brain-gut relationship is highly connected to emotional health, and there is a proven connection between stress and anxiety and gut disorders such as Crohn's and IBS. This system governs a huge part of our health, so taking time to respect our bodies while we nourish them is so, so, so important.

- Also, if we are engaging in self-loathing for eating the dark-chocolate, peanut butter mousse, there is a decent chance it isn't being digested with ease. Whenever possible, we want mind-body synergy. We are one being; nothing is separate, and certainly our emotions are not separate from our physical bodies. If we are loving up on the mousse and expressing gratitude for the opportunity to enjoy it, both the mind and body can accept this pleasure. In an ideal world, said mousse is made with beautiful ingredients by someone who loves his or her trade and has infused it with good prana (life force). But as we noted earlier, life isn't always ideal, so we make choices with intention, awareness, and respect toward our bodies. The ninety-nine cent vanilla cone may not be organic, but the person who served it to you may have scooped it with pride and care and smiled when she presented it to you. This too is a form of prana.

73

- Infusing food with prana starts from step one. Connect with your food while you choose it at the store, while you prepare it, and definitely while you eat and digest it. Notice the changes in your overall food experiences when you introduce this practice. And notice if this in turn connects you with Source and nature.

- Juicing for me is king. Well, actually, queen, because I'm a woman. I am not going to say you need to go out and buy a $400 juicer and turn into a crazy juice lady. I mean, I think crazy juice ladies are special and I swear by my juice, but I said I'd keep it simple. Juicing is a powerful way to feed our cells. I often hear mine making slurping sounds when I drink a jar of freshly made juice. Some say fresh juice has too much sugar and not enough fibre. To that I say BS. I've been juicing for nearly thirty years. Omg! It has yet to have a negative effect on my body. That said, I stay away from juicing tons of sweet vegetables or fruits. As a rule, I juice vegetables like celery, cucumber, beets. (Sweet, yes, but one beet for a whole juice juiced with other non-sweet vegetables works for me, and beets are an amazing tonic and blood cleaner.) I also like cabbage, radishes, and bitter greens like dandelion, and I stick to vegetables with higher water content versus, kale for example. To add some bit of sweetness, I will often add an apple, and for some zing and cleansing properties, always a lemon. It just makes everything pop. Additional gems are fresh ginger, turmeric, or even garlic when you need a real immune boost. I drink it immediately or if need be store it in a tightly sealed jar in the fridge, but ninety-nine percent of the time I drink it right away. After years of practice, I have managed to complete the whole process in under eight minutes from fridge to clean up. I use a centrifugal-style juicer, which is great for hard fruits and vegetables like the ones listed above. There are juicers specific for greens, which don't generate any heat during the process and thus are said to be better for preserving the nutrients, but frankly they do take a lot more time to prep i.e. lots of chopping, as the chute is much smaller and it's much more time-consuming to clean the multiple components, so I stick to my basic one. I have been using the same one since 2012 and it serves me just fine!

- Minimize too many food combinations. Ever notice how when you eat many things at once, your belly is like, "um, yeah no." Fruit as a rule is most easily digested on its own, not after a heavy consumption of food or when combined with other things. That whole "eat dinner and then have some fruit for dessert" is about as mean to your belly as you can get. Eat your fruit thirty minutes before other foods, or at least an hour after so that it doesn't sit there on top of other foods and ferment while it waits its turn. It is digested easily, so why get in the way of it by mixing it with heavy protein or dairy. It isn't a must, but it certainly is a way to be kind to your body. Again, this is just from personal experience.

- I feel better when I combine carbohydrates with vegetable, or protein with vegetables, but less awesome when I combine protein and carbohydrates. Unless it is in the form of a protein shake or smoothie that has all of these components. Shakes are good to have on hand for complete and balanced nourishment when I'm on the go or feeling like a nice boost of clean protein that tastes awesome, is quick, and can sustain me for a few hours. I choose shakes that are made with organic protein powder, no added sweeteners, definitely no artificial ingredients or corn syrups, and that are nourishing and easy to digest.

- Avoid refined sugar whenever possible. We have heard that white processed sugar is more addictive than heroin. Whether or not that is entirely true is not something I can comment on with a hundred percent certainty or irrefutable facts. I know people who try to "get off" sugar have a helluva time, which says something. What we do know is that refined sugar is responsible for or contributes heavily to mood swings, headaches, suppression of the immune system, obesity, inflammation, and many other conditions resulting in dis-ease. I for one, eat dark chocolate every day. Yes, every single day. It contains sugar, albeit a small amount, which is usually in the form of coconut sugar or a raw, unprocessed sugar but is sugar nonetheless. I am not saying I am perfect. I am saying that avoiding refined and processed sugars will positively impact your health, and when you do consume sugar, consider the source and kind. In addition to the obvious negative impacts on our bodies, sugar messes with our brain, which governs the body, so it contributes to mood swings, energy crashes, and quite literally makes us crazy. Life is crazy enough; we don't need any help there. Stay away from sugar as often as you can and then stand back and watch your life change.

- Minimize simple carbs. I am not a nutritionist, remember, and I know carbs have their place and purpose in our overall balanced health. They are crucial for performance in certain forms of exercise, and they keep our brain happy. I'm simply saying that as a rule I don't eat a lot "heavy" carbs like breads, pasta, rice, or crackers made from rice, corn, or otherwise. I tend to get mine in the form of root vegetables, and when I'm feeling particularly carb-deprived, I will have a bigass bowl of popcorn made on the stove, drenched in coconut oil and butter, and seasoned with sea salt, chili powder, black pepper and occasionally nutritional yeast. I will get into this a bit in the next section because there are ways to eat in accordance with the seasons, thus optimizing what is available, local, and fresh. Summer is a dry season, so it's not typically ideal to consume dry foods, for example popcorn, but when we add "wet" or "heavy" components like coconut oil or ghee (clarified butter), we transform that dry food into a nourishing, heavier, wetter food and then it becomes seasonally appropriate.

- According to Ayurveda, there are six tastes: sweet, sour, salty, bitter, astringent, and pungent. Incorporate the six tastes into every meal and you will be shocked with how satiated and nourished you feel. When we include these in every meal, we create a sense of balance so that we aren't left with extreme cravings. Below is a list of these six tastes, found from a basic Ayurveda search online, and examples of the foods that fit into each category.

Sweet:
- Most grains such as wheat, rice, barley, and corn
- Pulses (legumes), such as beans, lentils, and peas
- Milk and sweet milk products such as ghee, cream, and butter
- Sweet fruits (especially dried) such as dates, figs, grapes, pear, coconut, and mango
- Cooked vegetables such as potato, sweet potato, carrot, beetroot, cauliflower, and string beans
- Sugar in any form such as raw, refined, brown, white, molasses, and sugar cane juice

Sour:
- Sour fruits such as lemon, lime, sour orange, sour pineapple, passion fruit, sour cherries, plum, and tamarind
- Sour milk products such as yogurt, cheese, whey, and sour cream
- Fermented substances (other than cultured milk products) such as wine, vinegar, soy sauce, or sour cabbage
- Carbonated beverages (including soft drinks or beer)

Salty:
- Any kind of salt such as rock salt, sea salt, and salt from the ground
- Any food to which salt has been added

Pungent:
- Spices such as chili, black pepper, mustard seeds, ginger, cumin, cloves, cardamom, and garlic
- Mild spices such as turmeric, anise, cinnamon, and fresh herbs such as oregano, thyme, and mint
- Raw vegetables such as radish, onion, and cauliflower

Bitter:
- Vegetables such as chicory and bitter gourd; other green leafy vegetables such as spinach, green cabbage, and brussels sprouts
- Fruits such as olives, grapefruit, and cocoa
- Spices such as fenugreek and turmeric

Astringent:
- Turmeric, honey, walnuts, and hazelnuts
- Pulses such as beans, lentils, peas
- Vegetables such as sprouts, lettuce, and other green leafy vegetables; most raw vegetables
- Fruits such as pomegranate, berries, persimmon, rose, apple, and most unripe fruits

Once a month, give your digestion a break. Take a load off. Consume easy to digest, clean foods like juice, broth soup, and lightly steamed vegetables, and avoid harder to digest and heavy foods like meat, cheese, and even nuts, unless they are soaked in advance. Keep it simple. If it helps to put this into context, imagine you had food poisoning the night before. How would you eat the next day? How kind would you be to your digestive system? Be that kind. Better yet, be that kind most of the time. The more we give our system to digest, the harder it has to work, and the less energy it has to optimize other bodily functions. The body likes simplicity. How do you like answering the phone, talking to your toddler, cooking, having the TV on in the background, and answering your other kid's homework question while thinking about what time you have to leave to get to your doctor's appointment on time and which traffic route to take because you just heard that construction is now on your regular route. If you're like me and you don't have kids, replace that scenario with your own reality. You get my point. Simplify and give your body a break once in a while.

Bottom line: our digestive systems are working hard for us almost all the time because we tax them, often. We give them a lot of food all at once, in stimulating environments, which impacts our emotional and mental state while we are eating, and we do this several times a day. We are complex beings, yes, but our brains and bodily systems prefer simplicity, because their jobs are already complex enough. Your body works for you. Help it. Care for it. Nourish it. Be kind to it. Respect it. Eat slowly. Mindfully. Enjoy your food, either alone or with company you enjoy. Give thanks. If you aren't doing any of these things on a semi-regular basis, rather than judging yourself, consider introducing them. Close your eyes. Feel your belly, feel your body and ask it what it needs. Apologize to it if you need to. Accept. Breathe new life into your being and carry on.

SOAPBOX TIME

What you get is what you read. It's all there.

Here's where you might not love me ... but remember ... I'm passionate and I want to support you.

Sometimes we consume things that we don't even know are present in our food, and we wonder why we feel lethargic, bloated, or even nervous and anxious. I have been a label reader for the majority of my life. In this day and age, it is must.

Not reading the ingredient labels and pretending some of the ingredients are not harmful is like closing your eyes before you cross the street for fear you may see the cars coming. It's ludicrous and dangerous. Read read read, and then make an informed decision. And please please please do the same for your kids. They will eat things other than goldfish crackers and cheese strings if those things are no longer options for them. They trust us to feed and nourish them, let's do our jobs.

EXPENSIVE VS. INVESTMENT

Back in 2000, I shared my passion for wellness while away at school on a student's budget. Even though I was broke-ish financially, I lived my truth. I still bought organic food, just less of it, practiced yoga, and juiced my heart out. There is a myth that healthy living is expensive, and don't get me started on that word. If you want something, you'll pay anything for it. If it has value. If it doesn't, you won't, but that doesn't mean it is expensive. It means it isn't important or relevant or valuable to you. Living a vibrant, glowy life doesn't have to be expensive. I earn less now than I have at many points in my life, yet I feel my healthiest … it's curious, huh? Health isn't about money.

Yes, food costs, but you're already buying food, so it's simply a redirect of those same resources. When you choose to see food as an investment, it takes on new energy. Over time it may even feel inexpensive, like worth every cent and more, because the impact on your life and health is so extensive, you stop caring about what it costs financially and instead start asking what is the cost of not eating this way. You may get more creative with food and waste less. Who knows?

Perhaps you don't ask any questions, you don't overthink, and you are simply living life, enjoying your health while not needing to justify anything, and definitely not looking back. Not to mention you are spending less on quick fixes like antacids, heartburn medication, and other pharmaceuticals that put Band-Aids on our digestive ailments.

Congratulations, you passed the first soap box test! Hope you're still with me.

REAL LIFE EXAMPLE

When I was about twenty-five, I moved to Calgary. I lasted a month. I went there out of some kind of not-sure-what-to-do-with-my-life-ness, and got a job as a server. Walked in, rocked my interview, but stunk miserably at the actual serving part, proceeding to get so anxious about failing and pissing off all the impatient servers, who clearly didn't appreciate having the opportunity to light the way for newbies and instead huffed and puffed while I stood there at the menu screen entering my orders, that I stopped showing up, and spent the rest of the month eating chocolate and crying. I came home twenty pounds heavier. Literally. One month—twenty pounds. I had struggled with body image and binge eating before, but this was different. I was probably on the verge of actually being depressed. I was what I ate, and nothing fuels a depressed mindset more than gaining weight and feeling sluggish and like a failure. I moved back home. I started moving again. I started back on my juice, and within a few weeks, excess weight released and I was on my way "back" and forward to my wonderful self. We are what we eat. I was primarily made up of sugar and fat at that time, and I felt miserable. Food has the power to heal or harm. I had not been kind to my temple. I started to become my anxiety and fears. I had not yet learned that I was actually the one in charge of them, and so I let them take charge. When I started to fuel my body, raise my frequency through my food, and revisit the practices that I knew for the most part helped me feel strong, vital, and energetic, I bounced back relatively quickly and easily. Food is powerful. Either way. And everything is relative. Sometimes we need to feel like crap so that we can fully appreciate how blessed we are to have the choice to feel better.

NEXT SOAPBOX
YES, ALREADY.

Treat can be defined as *provide someone with (food, drink, or entertainment) at one's own expense,* or—and this is the relevant one for this purpose— *an event or item that is out of the ordinary and gives great pleasure.*

Somewhere along the way this turned into weekend hedonism and sabotaging our wellness by way of excessive alcohol, sweets, and giant brunches, and justifying it all in the name of "I deserve to treat myself." Kinda like Vegas.

When we say we are giving ourselves a treat, is that our way of truly giving our bodies what they need, or is it a cop-out and a way to please our minds because we are craving sugar and confusing our emotional needs with our physiological needs? Are you indulging because you hate your job, and so the first Friday evening after a hellish week warrants a treat? Are you feeling overwhelmed from taking care of everyone in your family, feeling unappreciated, depleted, and perhaps sorry for yourself, and so you're going to comfort yourself with a bottle of wine or eat that bag of cheetos? Have you overindulged in drinks and the best way to recover is to gorge yourself to sop up the excess alcohol? There are many reasons why humans overdo it when it comes to food. And hey, I am the first one to love up on some dark chocolate or even a peanut-buster parfait on the odd occasion. I have spent many years eating emotionally, and so now when I eat something I really desire, I know why. Where is your desire coming from? Is it a physiological need or an emotional one? Remember, I don't know all the answers I am just posing the questions, no judgment. Here's where I invite you to get curious. You are the only one you need to answer to. And as I've invited you to do all along, keep it real, be honest.

RECAP

—

Eat clean, fuel your body with food that is alive, give your digestion a break, eat when you're hungry not when you're not, and remember that how we eat is as important as what we eat. Gratitude, positive mindset, and intention are important parts of our mental diet. Your body is the only place you have to live. You want to be wild and enjoy the pleasure of life, so keep your body at its most vibrant, resilient, and healthy. It will thank you.

SIMPLICITY

This page is short 'n sweet for a reason.

Simple living is so liberating. There is a reason I have the Sanskrit word "moksha" tattooed on my arm. It means liberation, and in life I choose as many liberating practices, behaviours, relationships, and interactions as I can. Plain and simple.

When I go on a holiday, I take a carry-on, whether it is for two-days or eighteen. I like walking off a plane and going. Waiting is borrrring.

I do things myself.

I don't solicit a team of people to make decisions or to help me move.

I use mason jars for glasses.

I own three appliances: a juicer, a Magic Bullet, and an espresso machine.

I like life to be:

> As easy as possible.
>
> Uncomplicated.
>
> Drama-free—don't underestimate the power of this one.

And guess what. That's exactly the life I've built. You may want something different, and that's your choice.

I've had things, and lots of them; I've had luxuries. I've been involved in people's lives and have had them involved in mine, and I have found my most easeful and content days have been when I've had the least amount of stuff and the most amount of stillness, quiet, and opportunity for introspection. I still spend time with people and enjoy nice things. I am inviting you to consider that the more you have, whether it is stuff, relationships, commitments, or plans, the greater the opportunity for complexity to worm its way in, and the less opportunity for ommmmm.

What does living simply have to do with releasing your Inner Wild? Not sure it does, but it is something I do and something I believe wholeheartedly contributes to my happiness and wholeness. And maybe it frees up more time to get Wild. Hehe.

Where and what can you simplify? What can you purge, physically and energetically? What one step can you take to clear some crap and make space?

NO RECAP REQUIRED.

BE A-OK WITH NUMERO UNO

One of the most important lessons I have learned in this life is how to be OK with who I am. When I say OK, I mean totally OK, like satisfied and cool with it. I don't know about you, but I love and appreciate time to myself. Eating, sleeping, cooking, cleaning, listening to music... in many cases, although certainly not all, these things are often done with a partner, offspring, roommate, or parent. Spending time with another or several others can be a gift indeed. It is also a gift to practice spending time with your solo self, and I'm talking minus the phone and other means of communication. How comfortable are you really with who you are? How comfortable are you in your skin? Are you comfortable going out to dinner alone? I am not suggesting it is wrong to not feel comfortable. Heck, some people just don't enjoy dining alone, but it is often due to a fear of the perception of others. Will people think I'm a "loser" if I eat alone? Who will I talk with? What do I do with the time between ordering and eating? My invitation to you is to take yourself out. Sit alone. Take in the sights, smells, and sounds. Enjoy your food. Be with yourself and see how you like it. If you enjoy it, great! If you don't, also great, or there may be some work still to do so that you get to a point where you can be alone with your thoughts without needing a distraction or wanting to jump out of your skin. It is a pretty important life skill to be OK with who you are and to even enjoy your own company. On the plus side, it's good for digestion to eat without blabbing or being distracted.

See, you are a magical human being with unique skills, talents, and gifts. When you start to spend more time alone and get to know yourself more intimately without the interruption or barrage of opinions, projections, and judgments, you will begin to see and appreciate your own company, which in my opinion will make the being OK with being solo even easier. Then when we spend time with other people, it's almost like those moments are bonuses. Does that make sense? Rather than using those times (consciously or otherwise) to be validated, boosted, praised, distracted, or entertained, we can enjoy those moments with others so fully, knowing inside that we are just perfect as we are—that we don't need anything. There is a certain freedom and ease that then fills the space.

RECAP

—

Learn to be OK with #1. I can say with confidence your life will become more joyful when you start enjoying your own company. It becomes even sweeter when you know how amazing you truly are. You may even start bumping other people in order to plan date nights with yourself.

FIND YOUR TRIBE AND A FAN CLUB

————

Fab Five

"Anyone I allow to enter my magical world needs to be a catalyst to my dreams." I read this on my social media feed. It was a share by an essential-oils lover. Loved it! Sharin' it!

We've all heard that we are like the five people we spend the most time with. Who are your fab five? Here is a reminder to have a look without judgment. Get curious. How do you feel around these people? Do you laugh and sparkle? Do you feel free and safe? Do you feel you can accomplish anything?

Are you on guard and defensive? Do you shrink in their presence?

Are your fab five catalysts to your dreams?

These are things to notice, because guess what … this is very likely who you will start to emulate.

Do you have five people you can name? If you are noticing you don't have five close people in your life, or that the five you have aren't who you want to be most like, don't fret. Notice. Decide who you want your tribe to be in accordance with your needs, characteristics, and qualities, and then go seek and find them.

I'll admit I'm kind of a lone, wild wolfette, which is not the greatest thing according to studies that show who lives the longest and why, i.e. those who belong to a community. But I do have deep, meaningful connections with people, just not tons. I am social and I also love my quiet personal time where I can recharge and be free to be exactly how I want to be. Connecting with other souls is important, and actual human connection is critical to our emotional and mental well-being. If you are like me, AKA this weirdo blend of intro and extra-vert, I believe it is particularly important to pay attention to your fab five. Be discerning about who you let into your physical and mental space.

Take a pause: write down your fab five. Examine the people who you spend the most time with. Ask yourself if they are healthy for you or if you need to re-evaluate. No judgment, just do the exercise. Stay in the curious mind.

FAN CLUB!

Next, consider who you can crown to be your biggest fan, your running mate. This can be a partner or lover but doesn't have to be. This is someone who wants nothing more than to see you succeed in the wildest of ways.

These people exist, I swear! Find someone with whom you can share your deepest fears, to whom you can expose yourself. When we open up to being critiqued and challenged because we know it is all coming from a place of love with our best interest at heart, then we know we've found our fan. When we let down our guard, toss the ego, and let in the light of the people whom we trust fully and deeply, we can use what they've offered for our highest good, which is in turn also for the highest good of the Universe. You can use that vulnerability toward your personal growth to become even more awesome and then support others on their paths to being awesome too.

I have a fan. I didn't ask for one with my words, but my actions proved otherwise. I requested one in subtle ways and then, lo and behold, I was granted one. I knew I needed someone to love and guide my Wild nature. Not in a controlling way, but in a stay-on-track-woman you have so much to offer the world, I love you, now get 'er done, kind of way. The Universe hears our thoughts, words, and actions and responds in kind. It even hears our whispers, because although we may not shout it out, when the wishes and desires are so strong, they carry with them a loud energy.

I have never been so much in awe of my life as I have been these last two years. I am beyond blessed. I have the incredible opportunity to have the company of some of the most extraordinary people. I am amazed daily by the people who continue to share their limited time with me, to shower me with their love, protect me with their sacred Spirit connections, and watch over me from above like eagles watching over their nests.

You might be thinking, *Oh good for her. I don't know anyone like that and my "fab five" aren't so fab*. Guess what. Mine weren't always either. There were times when the people I spent time with sucked my life force or dimmed my shine. I spent time with people who, while they were wonderful in many ways, were not necessarily good *for* me or the people I wanted to be most like, and so I changed my circumstance. So can you. It doesn't have to be overnight, although it can be. Doesn't have to mean cutting all your people out, although it can. It doesn't have to mean actively hunting for your fab five, but it can. You are the decision maker of your own life. Do what you need to do to ensure your happiness.

Invite your tribe in by creating space either by letting something or someone go or simply by making the choice that you want more amazing people in your circle.

I am suuuuper selective about what I share and with whom. Sometimes people think that because I am a yoga teacher I always have it together, that I have not been through adversity, emotionally excruciating times, weight gains and losses, panic attacks, times where I questioned my self-esteem, and all the regular stuff that everyone goes through in life... I may not always share publicly but I have my tribe and I believe fully in the importance of being able to connect with people I trust, love and appreciate.

When you find people with whom you can share your story, and not just the shiny, sparkly parts, then you know you've found your people. Your tribe. There is something so comforting about this. There is no need to rush to find them because they will present themselves at the perfect time, and when they do, you will simply know.

RECAP

—

Choose wisely. Know that your tribe may very well change over time and that's perfect. Stay open to who might enter your life and what they have to offer.
Some people will bless your life in such ways you may even question whether you deserve it. Trust me, you do.

THE DIVINE FEMININE

The Divine feminine: here is where your Wild, ancient, earthy woman also dwells.

What is the Divine feminine? you ask. The words "Divine," "goddess," "Divine feminine," get tossed around a lot, don't they? We use them without truly understanding what they mean. Kinda like the word "Wild" or "badass" (smile).

Most people associate the word "goddess," which literally means female deity, and the phrase "Divine goddess," to be some kind of woman's right to be worshipped. Snapping our fingers like Beyoncé in one of her *Boy, you don't deserve me* type songs, and flipping our hair, to the left, to the left, a Divine goddess does not make. The Divine feminine is actually a quality that lives within both our feminine and masculine selves. It represents the connection to the part of us that nurtures, the part of us that is empathic and intuitive. Creativity, community, and all sensuality lie within the Divine feminine. Is the Divine feminine energy, sometimes known as shakti, something to be honoured and worshipped? Hell yeah. Buuuut, we need to do the work to earn that, we don't get praised just because we are women. We must do the work, find our shakti, embrace it, and at the same time recognize it in others, including men who connect to their feminine energy.

Perhaps you know your Divine Wild woman very intimately, or perhaps you still have yet to explore her. Perhaps you have an idea about her needs and wants but haven't connected with her closely enough to understand her fully. Perhaps, even though you're a woman, you operate from the masculine energy the majority of the time. In a busy world, it is our masculine energy that rules most daily tasks, business, and decision-making. It is the logical, action-oriented side of us that gets shit done. We are not really taught how to make decisions from our feminine energy, and so it is no wonder most people are not in touch with this energy at all, or at the very least have an energy imbalance.

Any and all of this is perfectly OK. It is my hope and prayer, as I said at the start of this book, that along your own personal, intimate, and unique journey, you discover and rediscover your Divine Wild woman. Women were the primal healers, the shamans, the caregivers, and the sustainers of families. To be a woman is no light responsibility. My invitation to you is to step into the role, own your feminine strength, and reconnect with your primal, Divine, goddess-like nature so that your Wild woman can emerge, fully.

In order to become one with her and to fully embrace her, first you need to meet her, like truly meet her. Sit down with her, have tea, have a chat, or many chats, and start to relearn her ways so that you may begin to understand what nourishes her. Ask her what her ancient self needs, to live in accordance with the seasons and the elements, with the current reality, which may be far from wild and more like a cubicle in a corporate office. Get real with your Divine feminine Self and, like you did with your Inner Wild, stay curious, get intimate, and connect. Take her to bed; ask her about her wildest dreams.

How can you connect to this shakti energy? One of the most important and significant ways to connect with our feminine energy is through our cycles, our moon time. How we prepare and move within the flow of our moon cycle is how, in essence, we move through life, because it is in accordance with nature, the moon, and the seasons that our moon cycle ebbs and flows. As this cycle repeats, so do our patterns and ways of being.

Each week within our cycle, we as women—and moreoever, conscious women who are aware of our cycles—often move through very real, very deep, and very significant shifts. We can go from feeling creative and alert, energized and motivated, to introspective, withdrawn, or even depressed, to a whole host of other emotions in between. This complex nature is often oversimplified and, frankly, belittled as hormonal, erratic, and crazy. It may be hormone-related, but don't ever let anyone tell you that what you experience or what becomes heightened or more intense throughout this cycle is anything less than beautiful, true, and deserving of respect. If we aren't careful, we can chalk up some of our most brilliant, creative thoughts, ideas and visions to PMS or "being a woman who isn't thinking straight" because members of society have shrunk our magnificence down to a time of the month, often ridiculed and associated with negativity. Protect your moon time, honour and celebrate it. Connecting with this cycle and all of its glory can be the difference between feeling out of sorts, out of place, and out of our minds to feeling creative, highly intelligent, intuitive, and practicing self-care.

Another way I like to honour my Divine feminine (and this may seem odd, so take it or leave it), is to spend time with Sacred Masculine energy, as I believe this can help us to recognize and even more clearly identify our Divine feminine. Not only can it assist an otherwise highly masculine person, male or female, to become softer, not weaker, softer, it can also cultivate our feminine energy on an ongoing basis so that we don't get complacent or forgetful, neglecting our Divine feminine.

As another brilliant saying goes:

I am woman hear me roar.

HERE'S WHERE I'M GONNA GET REAL STRAIGHT WITH YOU... YES, EVEN STRAIGHTER

Whatchoo waiting for? Life is now. As I said earlier, get out of your own way.

Every opportunity that I have taken on my path toward creating the life I wanted, I've carved out. Yes. From the first job I ever had to this moment right here, I have decided what it is that I wanted and I made it happen. Sometimes it took months, or years, and sometimes it took one phone call.

For the more challenging stuff, it depended on how badly I wanted it and what I was willing to do to get it. It required staying in the flow and knowing when to let go and when to watch things unfold. You might be thinking, *Well, I'm not like that. I don't call up random people and create my opportunities.*

Here's what I say to that: What you want, you can have. You need to decide how badly you want it. If you are not living the life you want, it is simply because you haven't made the choices necessary to make it happen. Obligations, jobs, families, aging parents, financial "woes" are all excuses that you can tell yourself are the reasons you aren't where you want to be.

I could go on and on about the things I wanted and how I went about creating the opportunities to get them and was not thrown off course by the numerous times I was told "no" or "later" or "that won't work" or "you're crazy." I could have let those be the last times I tried. I could have let a "no" to my proposal to write for a magazine I wanted to write for end with that first no. A year later, I was one of the top writers, was asked to edit, and was given assignments interviewing celebrities. We simply won't know where life will take us if we settle for mediocrity and let someone else's perceptions of possibility become our truths.

What do you want in this lifetime, and what will it take to get it? What are you willing to do to get what you want?

Stop delaying and start creating it. It's time to get off your butt, get Wild, and make stuff happen. Life is happening now. I say all of this out of my deepest desire for you to rise to your highest potential, to be your happiest and healthiest and because I know that with hard work it is all possible.

Get out of your own way for once and see what is on the other side of your fears. What's the worst that will happen? You won't get the job, you won't lose the weight, your date won't work out? Who cares!!?!? I'd dare to argue the opposite of those things will probably happen, and along the way the lessons you will learn will be instrumental in whatever it is that you choose to do next.

I want you to take a good, hard look at yourself and ask, "Where can I step up? Where can I show up? How can I show up differently in order to create my best life? Am I giving this life my all"? Even if you don't make a monumental shift today, do something, any-thing, to step outside your comfort zone and start creating the life you want. The worst that will happen is it won't work. Again, who cares?? At least you tried. Then dust off and try again. And again. And again.

I used to look at people who had what I wanted (freedom, strength, confidence) and think *I don't know if I can ever have that. I'm not like that. I don't have that skill.* And whatever other self-limiting belief that was "true" for me at the time.

I've experienced doubt many times in my life, but I've never dwelled. I got to work. Of course it takes work that you need to be willing to do, and the reward is astounding.

Stop complaining about how "crazy busy" life is, how you take care of everyone else, how you're overwhelmed. No one cares. I say that in the most sensitive way I can. No one cares.

I had no idea the degree to which I'd be rewarded with the opportunity to create exactly the life I desired once I started doing what I'm really good at, trusting my worth, getting out of my way, having some faith, knowing my gifts, and trusting my Inner Wild to lead me in the right direction. Life rewards risk, remember? Life rewards action.

Get this … the best thing about the story I'll share in a moment is that for a year or maybe more, I secretly prayed for a layoff from that "great" job I mentioned earlier. Not because I didn't want to work, but because I knew I was destined for something bigger, and because, layoffs rock. I mean who doesn't want to get paid for not working? I didn't want to be fired, of course, or to quit until I had a safety net, because I had a mortgage to pay and a lifestyle to support. But in the back of my mind and occasionally to my then-partner, I'd wish for a layoff just until I could figure out the next step. Well, on the day I was granted my wish in January of 2015, I was reminded that even if we forget about our wish temporarily, what we put out there has its way of showing up. Exactly when, we don't know. I worked hard all of my days at that job. I gave it my all and was never ungrateful. I also knew it wasn't for me anymore, and so I was building my future in other ways. It was like my higher intelligence knew a transition was coming. I may have stopped obsessing over the layoff, but the intention had already been set in motion, and so it went.

I had made wonderful contacts on a small island near where I currently live, which is about five hours from Vancouver. I started spending more and more time there. When the time came for me to leave Vancouver, I had a safe place to go. A refuge, a community. This all transpired over three years, and it was like somewhere in the ethers, my message had been heard and I was building my safe haven. I lived there for almost two years.

How was that created? Not totally consciously, but not totally unconsciously either. It wasn't like I was even aware that I was building this safety net, because at the time I could not have imagined being laid off or my relationship ending … hmmm. Yet somehow my request for a layoff and some kind of change was heard.

I believe in the notion "everything in its own time." There is also a fine line between letting this happen in its "own time" and manifesting, growing, and making it happen. The fun part is that we never really know until we do it. Is it time? Is it too early, too late?

Fear is tricky, because it can keep us safe and protected in a good way, but it can also keep us small and stuck if we aren't careful and if we linger there. If we aren't strong enough in the mind, we can be tricked by fear into believing we need to stay small and safe and stuck. We move when the time is "right," and sometimes it's hard to know when that is. On occasion we are not exactly on time for moving ahead and then we get to experience what comes along with that. Sometimes we get impatient and we force things; other times we allow ourselves to become lazy or fearful and so we miss an opportunity. There is a time to shift gears, and it's important to know when. Too soon and it gets jerky, too late and we start to rev! Only we know when the time is right for us, and sometimes we have to risk it and see what's on the other side of fear. Often, we experience freedom on the other side.

Then there is the notion that we are always exactly where we need to be. I agree. What I also know is that there comes a point when we simply need to decide. We need to take charge of our lives and choose, stay, go, here, there, yes, no. The more often we choose versus being the recipient of others' choices and decisions, the more comfortable we become trusting our intuition and higher intelligence. And then, the less scary it feels, so the more we do it, the higher we climb, the more we rock the hell outta life! Next thing you know, people are asking how you got to where you are.

My answer to that questions is always: Choice by choice by choice.

During my time living on that small island, I reached a point where I was stuck. I didn't want to stay, but I had nowhere to go. For about six months I drifted, couch surfed, stayed with relatives for a week here or there, visited Mom and Dad here and there, rented places for short-term stints here and there. Forty-two and couch surfing ... greeeeeat. Not exactly where I thought I'd be at that point in my life.

I was ready to use every cent to my name, RRSPs, savings, and then some, to start a new business just so I could delve into something that I thought was in my future. I wanted to teach yoga and had always dreamed of having a space.

For months, I read aloud to myself and wrote down my goal, which was to move to this town nearby.

I had been telling everyone I knew for those months that I was looking for a place to live. I also turned to a guide in my life. I asked for help. For prayer. I went on a week-long stay to Mexico to see Mom and Dad. (Yes, it's very handy having snowbirds for parents while having minor or major breakdowns). While I was there, I got a message from a friend, who said she thought she had found me a place and it had an empty garage below and perhaps I could use it for a studio. Vacancies in that town were pretty much non-existent, not to mention a space that I could convert into a yoga practice room. Boom!

I messaged the homeowners from Mexico and basically told them I'd take it without having so much as a sweet clue what it looked like, where it was, or even how much it was.

On my way home from Mexico, I stopped in to this town en route back to the small island. I met the owners, saw the suite above the empty garage space, and told them I was in. No overthinking. Just action.

And then I packed up my stuff (took a day or two), I moved in, and I got to work. For the next two years this was the home of Wild Pose Yoga, a sacred space where people came to practice yoga, build community, enjoy aromatherapy treatments and education, and where my gifts were shared as my service to others. A space where people came to release their Inner Wild. Yes.

This experience is a beautiful manifestation of love, trust, networking, and how when we put out there what we want, and then we let go, magic happens. When we come from a place of service, things have a way of unfolding beautifully.

So all of the chapters that brought you to this moment—chapters on trusting, letting go, visualizing, affirming, limiting self-limiting beliefs, being of service, having boundaries, speaking your truth, taking care of your temple—all converge at this intersection to create a new reality.

Passion and belief in ourselves take us to places unknown and unimaginable.

Clear the mental clutter and negativity from your mind. Choose. Take action. Decide what you want to bring in more of, make a mental note and then a physical note or hundreds of notes, and tell people—declare it! Close your eyes and paint a picture. Jump. Both feet in.

What does it look and feel like to have your wish as your reality? Feel it in every cell. Believe you are deserving of it and that it is in the works for you right now. Then sit back and trust the process. Let go of perfection and expectations.

Whatever you do or don't do, whatever you choose or don't choose, please, please, please for the love of all things chocolaty and caffeinated, love yourself along the way, because once you do, life becomes a hell of a lot easier and way more fun.

Whether things come "easily" or with more effort, either way, you are alive *now*, so why not use your time wisely to cultivate what will bring you a lifetime of peace, joy, health, passion, adventure, and Wild wonder!

It is time to dig deep. Reconnect with your Inner Wild. Who is she? How does she move? What are her ways? Who does she attract? Let her out and let her rule for a change. See where she takes you. Feed her. Love her. Respect her. Honour her. And trust her. She is you.

ABOUT THE AUTHOR

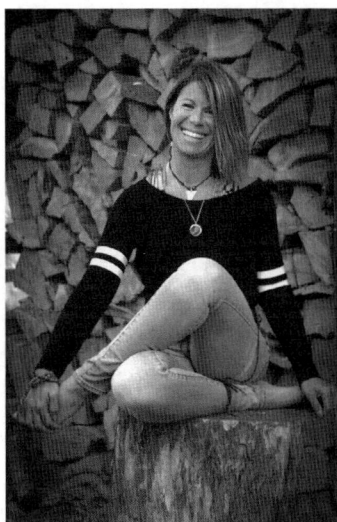

Dana Mahon has been a health and wellness champion since she was a teenager and has dedicated her life to this path ever since. For the past two decades Dana has studied and worked in the health and wellness industry, inspiring her to create and run two successful Yoga businesses, for adults and youth.

Dana's unwavering belief and experience is that when we honour all aspects of our well-being including speaking our truth and knowing our worth, we become more balanced, content and peaceful. Through her love of Yoga teaching, aromatherapy, and passion for natural living, Dana has supported hundreds of people on their wellness journeys.

She lives on the stunning West Coast of British Columbia on Vancouver Island. *Release Your Inner Wild* is her first book.

Read more about Dana at releaseyourinnerwild.com

10

Printed in Canada